Bucket Diagrams:
A Problem-Solving Approach
to Renal Physiology

Bucket Diagrams:
A Problem-Solving Approach
to Renal Physiology

Herbert F. Janssen

Texas Tech University Press
Lubbock, Texas

This book was set in Times and Helvetica and printed on recycled, acid-free paper that meets the guidelines for permanence and durability of the Committee on Production Guidelines for Book Longevity of the Council on Library Resources.

Manufactured in the United States of America

Library of Congress Cataloging-in-Publication Data
Janssen, Herbert F.
    Bucket diagrams : a problem-solving approach to renal physiology /
Herbert F. Janssen.
        p. cm.
    ISBN 0-89672-323-2 (alk. paper)
    1. Kidneys—Physiology—Programmed instruction. I. Title.
    [DNLM: 1. Kidney—physiology—programmed instruction. 2. Kidney—
secretion—programmed instruction. 3. Kidney Concentrating
Ability—physiology—programmed instruction. WJ 18 J35b 1993]
    QP249.J36 1994
    612.4'63—dc20
    DNLM/DLC
    for Library of Congress   93-29223
                                                                                    CIP

94 95 96 97 98 99 00 01 02 / 9 8 7 6 5 4 3 2 1

Texas Tech University Press
Lubbock, Texas 79409-1037 USA
800-832-4042

PREFACE

Understanding renal function can be a challenge to students. Basic knowledge must be coupled with the ability to analyze a variety of situations that apply to the concepts of glomerular filtration, renal clearance, reabsorption, secretion, and countercurrent multiplication, for example. Problem-solving skills are challenging for the student to learn and the professor to teach. The diagrams provided in this problem-based study guide were developed to make this teaching and learning process more productive for both parties. Concepts are presented in a format that allows students to address renal function from a logical approach.

Problem solving as the foundation of medical education is fast becoming the standard to which all other methods will be compared. In this educational setting, the student becomes an active participant rather than an inactive observer. The problem-solving approach to education can be traced back to ancient times. Confucius is credited with having said "I hear and I forget, I see and I remember, I do and I understand."

As with any journey, the trip through this study guide must start at the beginning. Starting the trip in the middle does not allow you to build the foundation that is necessary if the concepts are to be understood fully. Each section is prefaced with learning objectives and includes a detailed explanation of the concepts being covered. The examples provided in each section test your ability to achieve these objectives and understand the concepts. The correct solution and explanation follow each example. You will need to review material relevant to any question that is incorrectly answered. If the questions are answered correctly, you may proceed to the next section.

The first section on glomerular filtration presents very straight forward concepts. The second section discusses inulin excretion and builds on the material covered in the first. Understanding the concepts and completing the examples in these sections are crucial to your ability to understand the more complicated concepts related to reabsorption, secretion, and concentrating mechanisms that are presented in later sections.

Bucket diagrams were first developed as a teaching aid in a comparative animal physiology course. The success achieved at this level prompted additional use of the diagrams with allied health students, nursing students, medical students, and graduate students. The name "bucket diagram" was supplied by an unknown student in medical physiology. Despite being unsophisticated, it is descriptive and unforgettable.

ACKNOWLEDGMENTS

I would like to thank all the people who helped in the development of this text. They include Winnie Cammack and Kathy Wright for typing the manuscript, David Williams and Kerri Carter for graphics work, Carole Young for editing the manuscript, Marilyn Steinborn for typesetting, and the entire Texas Tech University Press for their assistance. Melton Welch and Lawrence Schovanec contributed much to the mathmatical understanding of glomerular filtration. I would also like to express my appreciation to the medical school students at Texas Tech University Health Sciences Center who offered critical comments that undoubtedly helped to improve the presentation of the material covered in the text. Various colleagues also provided helpful suggestions that contributed much to the final product. To these individuals, I offer a heartfelt thanks.

To my sons—Dusty and Ryan

CONTENTS

CONTENTS

• Urine Concentrating Mechanisms •

• Body Fluids •

• Corrections Section •

BASIC RULES

Unless indicated otherwise, the following rules apply.

- Try to evaluate each situation logically. Do not look for "trick questions." The purpose of the programmed text is to help you understand the material, not to play mind games.

- The stylistic nephron used in the bucket diagrams is intended to represent all the nephrons in both human kidneys.

- Some values are rounded off for ease in performing the mathematical calculations. This rounding obscures the problem that mass balance is not maintained in the calculation of renal plasma flow (RPF) and the extraction ratio. (Further explanation is found in the Corrections Section.)

- The values you are given to solve the examples might not be in the format you need. For example, you may be given the concentration of a compound when you need to know the flow rate. You can convert concentration to flow rate by using the conversion formulae given in the Definitions Section.

- It is well known that the kidney will spill glucose into the urine before the filtered load of glucose reaches transport maximum. This is referred to as splay. In the bucket diagrams, splay is not considered unless otherwise indicated. For example, we assume that no glucose is lost in the urine until the filtered load exceeds transport maximum. A similar assumption is made for secreted compounds such as PAH. (An explanation of this is found in the Corrections Section.)

- Renal plasma flow (RPF) is defined as all the plasma that enters the kidney. Effective renal plasma flow (ERPF) is defined as the plasma that passes through a functional nephron. RPF generally exceeds ERPF by 10-15%. For ease of computation, RPF is considered to equal ERPF. (An explanation of the difference between RPF and ERPF is found in the Corrections Section.)

- Many of the values given in the bucket diagrams cannot be obtained experimentally, even in the laboratory. In these exam-

1

ples, such values are estimations based upon our knowledge of renal function.

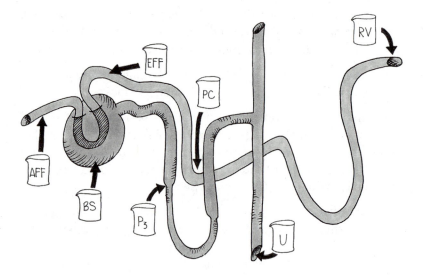

- The locations of the "buckets" are as follows:

  AFF = Afferent arteriole
  BS = Bowman's space
  EFF = Efferent arteriole
  P3 = End of the proximal tubule
  PC = Peritubular capillary across from the end of the proximal
            tubule
  RV = Renal vein
  U = urine

In the urine concentrating section several additional "buckets" are added to help identify more precisely the tubular sections of interest.

SYMBOLS

The following are used throughout the text, in the figures, and in the equations.

C_x — renal clearance of compound X. For example, C_{in} is the renal clearance of inulin.

CO — cardiac output

E_x — extraction ratio of compound X. For example, E_{in} is the extraction ratio of inulin.

$ERPF$ — effective renal plasma flow

FF — filtration fraction

GFR — glomerular filtration rate

G-T $balance$ — glomerulotubular balance

HCT — hematocrit

K_f — permeability of the capillary

$P1$ — early convoluted proximal tubule

$P2$ — late convoluted and early straight portion of the proximal tubule

$P3$ — final or straight portion of the proximal tubule

P_x — concentration of compound X in the plasma

Pa_x — concentration of compound X in the renal artery. This is equal to P_x or the concentration of the compound in a peripheral vein.

P_{BS} — hydrostatic (hydrolic) pressure in Bowman's space

P_c — hydrostatic (hydrolic) pressure in the capillary

Pv_x — concentration of compound X in the renal vein

π_{BS} — oncotic pressure in Bowman's space

π_c — oncotic pressue in the capillary

$\dot{Q}$ — volume of fluid/min (flow rate) in the Starling equation. This is the volume/min of fluid filtered across the capillary membrane.

Qe — quantity of a compound excreted per minute

Qf — quantity of a compound filtered per minute

RBF — renal blood flow

RF — renal fraction

RPF — renal plasma flow

3

Tm — transport maximum or the maximum amount per minute of compound that can be transported across the renal tubule

TF/P$_x$ — concentration of compound X in the tubular fluid (at a specific site) divided by the concentration of the compound in the plasma

U$_x$ — concentration of compound X in the urine

$\dot{V}$ — urine volume/min (flow rate)

DEFINITIONS

Clearance (C_x) is the volume of plasma that originally contained the amount of a solute excreted per minute. This volume is calculated by dividing the amount of a compound excreted per minute (Qe) by the plasma concentration (afferent arteriole concentration) of the compound. The amount of a compound that is excreted per minute is determined by multiplying the urine concentration of the compound (U_x) and the volume of urine found per minute ($\dot{V}$).

$$C_x = \frac{U_x \dot{V}}{P_x} = \frac{Qe}{P_x}$$

Conversion equations—Some of the values given in the examples in the text are not in a form that is useful to solve the examples. For example, the concentrate of a compound is given but you need the volume. The following equations should help.

$$\text{Amount} = \text{Concentration} \times \text{Volume} \qquad \text{Volume} = \frac{\text{Amount}}{\text{Concentration}}$$

$$\text{Concentration} = \frac{\text{Amount}}{\text{Volume}} \text{ or } \frac{\text{Amount/min}}{\text{Flow rate}} \qquad \text{Flow rate} = \frac{\text{Amount}}{\text{Concentration}}$$

$$\text{Amount/min} = \text{Concentration} \times \text{Flowrate}$$

Effective renal plasma flow (ERPF) is the plasma that flows through the functional nephrons. This value is usually considered to be 85-90% of renal plasma flow. (Note: In the bucket diagrams, ERPF is considered to be equal to renal plasma flow (RPF). This assumption ignores the 10-15% of plasma that enters the kidney but does not pass through a functional nephron. The difference is explained in the Corrections Section.)

Extraction ratio (E_x) is the amount per minute of a compound that is excreted divided by the amount per minute entering the afferent arteriole. In the clinical setting, this is calculated by dividing the difference between the plasma concentration and the renal vein concentration by the plasma concentration.

$$E_x = \frac{Pa_x - Pv_x}{Pa_x}$$

5

Filtered load is the amount per minute of a compound that appears in Bowman's space. For freely filtered compounds, filtered load is equal to glomerular filtration rate (GFR) times the plasma concentration of the given compound (P_X).

$$\text{Filtered Load} = \text{GFR} \times P_x$$

Filtration fraction (FF) is the glomerular filtration rate (GFR) divided by renal plasma flow (RPF). This is the percent of renal plasma that becomes glomerular filtrate per minute.

$$FF = \frac{GFR}{RPF}$$

Free-water clearance is defined as the volume of distilled water that would have to be added or subtracted from the volume of urine formed each minute to make the urine isosmotic with plasma. A negative free-water clearance indicates that a concentrated urine is being formed.

$$C_{H_2O} = \dot{V} - \frac{U_{Osm}\,\dot{V}}{P_{Osm}}$$

Where:

U_{Osm} = mOsm/kg H2O Concentration in the Urine
P_{Osm} = mOsm/kg H2O Concentration in the Plasma

Freely filtered describes the process by which compounds of low molecular weight cross the filtration barrier easily and appear in the filtrate at concentrations equal to the plasma concentration.

Glomerular filtration rate (GFR) is the rate at which fluid enters Bowman's space. This fluid is formed by the process of ultrafiltration through the glomerular capillaries. Glomerular filtration rate is calculated by determining the clearance of inulin.

$$GFR = C_{in} = \frac{U_{in}\,\dot{V}}{P_{in}}$$

Glomerulotubular balance (G-T balance) attempts to explain the observation that a relatively constant volume of glomerular filtrate is reabsorbed in the proximal tubule per minute. Normally, two-thirds of the filtered volume is reabsorbed; however, this can be altered by changes in hydration of the individual.

Isosmotic fluid reabsorption—The rate of fluid reabsorption in the proximal tubule is maintained so that the osmolality of the fluid does not change appreciably between Bowman's space and the end of the proximal tubule. This is largely due to the leaky epithelium of the proximal tubule, which allows water to be reabsorbed freely as various compounds are reabsorbed. The reabsorption of sodium has the greatest influence on the reabsorption of water in the proximal tubule.

Mass balance is a concept frequently used in chemical engineering. The concept requires that the amount/min of a solute and/or solvent entering a system must equal the amount that remains in the system and/or exits the system. For example, the flow rate of plasma entering the afferent arteriole must equal the flow rate of glomerular filtrate (GFR) plus the flow rate of plasma appearing in the efferent arteriole.

Milliosmole (mOsm)—1/1000 of a osmole or the amount of a substance that dissociates in water to form a millimole (mM) of active particles. A solution that contains a 1 mOsm concentration of active particles will exert a pressure equal to 19.3 mm Hg when dialyzed against distilled water across a semipermeable membrane.

Oncotic pressure is the osmotic pressure that can be attributed to colloid osmotic pressure (proteins) plus the alteration in equilibrium of ions caused by the Gibbs-Donnan effect. A description of this can be found in most renal text books.

Osmolality—The number of moles (gram equivalent weight) of an element or compound dissolved in one kilogram of water.

Osmolarity—The number of moles (gram equivalent weight) of an element or compound dissolved in enough solvent to give a total volume of one liter.

Osmole (Osm)—The amount of a substance that dissociates in water to form one mole of active particle. For example, one mole of glucose (which does not dissociate) yields one osmole when dissolved in water; however, one mole of sodium chloride produces two osmoles when placed in water and each NaCl molecule dissociates into Na^+ and Cl^-. In physiology, this is an important concept because of the effect particle concentration has on water movement. A solution that contains a 1 osmole concentration of active particles exerts a pressure equal to 19,300 mm Hg when dialyzed against distilled water across a semipermeable membrane.

Renal blood flow (RBF) is greater than renal plasma flow by the volume occupied by red blood cells. Renal blood flow is calculated by dividing renal plasma flow (RPF) by 1 minus the hematocrit (HCT).

$$RBF = \frac{RPF}{1 - HCT}$$

Renal fraction (RF) is defined as renal blood flow (RBF) divided by cardiac output (CO). Normally, the human kidneys receive 20-25% of cardiac output.

$$RF = \frac{RBF}{CO}$$

Renal plasma flow (RPF) is the volume of plasma that flows through the renal artery per minute. RPF is calculated by dividing the amount of a compound appearing in the urine per minute by the difference between the concentration of the compound in the renal artery and the renal vein. In the bucket diagrams, RPF is considered to equal the volume of plasma flowing through the afferent arterioles (instead of the renal artery) per minute. This ignores the 10-15% of plasma that normally enters the renal artery but does not pass by a functional nephron. A discussion of this is provided in the Corrections Section.

$$RPF = \frac{U_x \dot{V}}{Pa_x - Pv_x}$$

Splay—Normal human renal tubules reabsorb approximately 375 mg/min of filtered glucose (transport maximum). When the filtered load exceeds approximately 180 mg/min, some glucose appears in the urine, although the transport maximum for glucose has not been reached. This is an example of splay. Solute kinetics are thought to cause this phenomenon. Splay can also occur with secreted compounds. (Further explanation is given in the Corrections Section.)

Starling equilibrium equation—Named after E. H. Starling, the equation is used to calculate the rate of fluid movement across a membrane.

$$\dot{Q} = K_f [(P_C - P_t) - (\pi_C - \pi_t)]$$

In the kidney, the subscript "t" is often replaced by "BS" to signify Bowman's space.

TF/P$_x$ ratio is the concentration of compound X at various sites along the renal tubule divided by the concentration of the compound in the plasma passing through the afferent arteriole. This ratio can change as the compound moves along the tubule because of reabsorption or secretion of the compound or the reabsorption of water. (Remember the concentration of a compound in the afferent arteriole is considered to equal the concentration of the compound in any peripheral vein of the body.)

$$TF/P_x = \frac{Tubular\,concentration\,of\,X}{Pa_x}$$

Transport maximum (Tm) represents the maximum amount of a compound that can be secreted or reabsorbed by the renal tubules per minute. The following equations are applicable when the Tm has been exceeded. For reabsorbed compounds:

$$Tm = Filtered\ Load - amount/min\ excreted$$

For secreted compounds:

$$Tm = amount/min\ excreted - Filtered\ Load$$

GLOMERULAR CAPILLARY FILTRATION

Introduction

During the late 19th century, investigators debated the mechanisms involved in the formation of urine. One group lead by Ludwig held that a filtrate of plasma was formed in the glomerulus and that this was the initial process in the formation of urine. The opposing group, lead by Bowman and Heidenhain, maintained that urine was formed mainly by the process of tubular secretion. Starling addressed this question in a series of studies conducted near the turn of the century. In 1899 he published the results of several experiments designed to evaluate the effects of plasma proteins on filtration in the glomerulus. The importance of these studies has since extended far beyond its original intent. The equation that was developed based upon Starling's original work is now used to describe filtration in glomerular capillaries as well as capillaries throughout the body. The Starling equilibrium equation can be found written in several forms, a common version is:

$$\dot{Q} = K_f \left[(P_c - P_t) - (\pi_c - \pi_t) \right]$$

where:
$\dot{Q}$ = filtration rate
K_f = capillary permeability
P_c = hydrostatic pressure in the capillary
P_t = hydrostatic pressure in the tissue (or Bowman's space-P_{BS})
π_c = oncotic pressure in the interstitial space
π_t = oncotic pressure in the tissue (or Bowman's space- π_{BS})

The forces that determine glomerular filtration are the same as those that affect filtration in other capillaries throughout the body. Despite these similarities, several major differences exist.

First, the anatomy of the filtration barrier in the glomerular capillary is different from other tissues. The glomerular filtration barrier is highly permeable to small molecular weight compounds and highly impermeable to large molecules. The filtration barrier itself is negatively charged, making it impermeable to negatively charged particles. Particles with a positive charge cross the barrier easier than neutral or negatively charged particles of similar size and configuration. Large negatively charged particles are almost totally repelled by the glomerular filtration barrier. Proteins are in this latter group and are almost totally excluded from the entry into Bowman's space.

Second, the large cross-sectional area of the glomerular capillary provides not only a larger surface area for filtration but it also reduces resistance to flow along the length of the capillary. This means that capillary hydrostatic pressure does not decrease significantly along the length of the glomerular capillary as it does in a systemic capillary.

Third, the space surrounding the glomerular capillary is not filled with interstitial gel matrix and therefore does not have the same characteristics as a systemic capillary. In Bowman's space the hydrostatic pressure is usually greater than that found in the space around a systemic capillary.

Fourth, previously filtered fluid is not reabsorbed into the distal portion of the glomerular capillary as it is in a peripheral capillary. This occurs because, as mentioned above, glomerular capillary hydrostatic pressure does not decrease as the fluid moves along the length of the capillary. The maintenance of a higher pressure in the distal portion of the glomerular capillary allows a balance between the forces favoring filtration and those opposing filtration. The significance of this will be mentioned below.

Fifth, the fluid in a glomerular capillary passes through an arteriole on both ends of the capillary, whereas in a systemic capillary the fluid passes through an arteriole only before it enters the capillary. The double arteriole system in the kidney allows the flow rate along the capillary to be regulated independently of the hydrostatic pressure in the capillary.

Sixth, there is evidence that the permeability (K_f) of a glomerular capillary can be altered to change the glomerular filtration rate (GFR). It is thought that this regulation of K_f is achieved by the actions of angiotensin II on mesangial cells located between the glomerular capillaries.

Net filtration pressure is that pressure responsible for the formation of a glomerular filtrate and is the sum of the forces favoring and opposing the filtration process. Attempts have been made to esti-

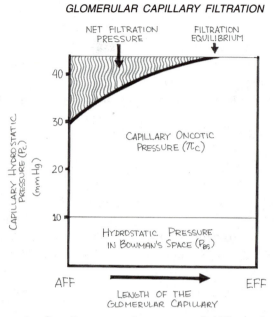

Figure 1. Oncotic pressure increases as fluid flows along the glomerular capillary. Filtration equilibrium is reached when the forces favoring filtration (P_C) and those opposing filtration ($P_{BS} + \pi_C$) are equal.

mate net filtration pressure in the kidney. The small size of a glomerular capillary makes the accuracy measurement of these pressures difficult, if not impossible, using currently available techniques. Despite these problems, estimations of these pressures have been made by knowledgeable investigators. Based upon these estimates, it is accepted that net filtration pressure is greatest near the afferent end of the capillary and decreases as the fluid moves toward the efferent end. Near the efferent end of the capillary filtration equilibrium (balance in the forces favoring and opposing filtration) is reached (Figure 1). Between this point and the efferent end of the capillary, no filtration occurs. This decrease in capillary filtration occurs because plasma oncotic pressure increases to offset the capillary hydrostatic pressure that favors filtration. The increase in plasma oncotic pressure occurs because the concentration of protein in the capillary rises as fluid is filtered from the plasma but protein is retained.

The examples that follow are intended to depict different conditions that occur if the afferent or efferent arteriole is constricted or dilated or the permeability of the filtration barrier is altered. Chang-

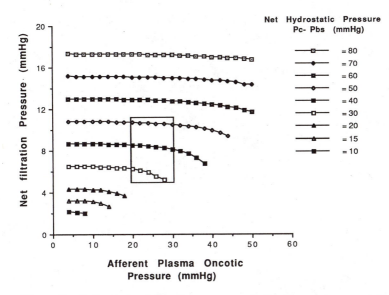

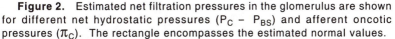

Figure 2. Estimated net filtration pressures in the glomerulus are shown for different net hydrostatic pressures (P_C – P_{BS}) and afferent oncotic pressures (π_C). The rectangle encompasses the estimated normal values.

ing hydrostatic pressure in the glomerular capillary by altering the vascular tone of the arterioles is part of the normal GFR regulation; however, changes in the glomerular hydrostatic pressure can be produced also by pathological conditions such as vascular disease (often secondary to diabetes mellitus) or blood clots in the vascular system. In addition to altering renal hemodynamics, many pathological conditions that produce renal complications involve alterations in the filtration barrier permeability (K_f). Most often these permeability changes are produced by the deposition of immune complexes on the basement membrane. Obviously, many variations in the filtration process can be produced by different pathological conditions. These many permutations are beyond the scope of this book.

In these examples, K_f is calculated based upon the assumption of a natural logarithmic increase in plasma oncotic pressure along the length of the glomerular capillary, with no decrease in capillary hydrostatic pressure. Figure 2 illustrates the different average net filtration pressures that would be expected under the various conditions.

When you are asked to determine a K_f value, use only the data in the table, not the value from the figure.

In each example you are asked to calculate several values needed to complete the table below the figure. The information needed to accomplish this task is provided and needs only your skills of logical deduction or simple math. The Starling equilibrium equation will be needed in all examples. Becoming intimately familiar with this equation will be of great value.

Objectives

- Explain and give examples showing how the Starling equilibrium equation can be used to calculate GFR.

- List factors that can alter capillary permeability in the kidney.

- Discuss why capillary permeability in the kidney may be greater for low molecular weight compounds but higher for proteins as compared to a skeletal muscle capillary.

- Explain what is meant by filtration equilibrium.

- Discuss how hydrostatic capillary pressure in the glomerulus can be altered by constriction or dilation of the afferent and efferent arterioles.

- Use the Starling equilibrium equation to explain how changing hydrostatic pressure in the glomerular capillary can change GFR independent of renal blood flow.

- Discuss the effects on filtration in a glomerular capillary if plasma oncotic pressure is increased or decreased.

- Explain the concept of K_f as used in the Starling equilibrium equation and show how changing this value can alter filtration.

- Calculate the missing values by using the Starling equilibrium equation and explain how each value is determined.

Example 1 – Altered K_f: Problem

INCREASED K_f DECREASED K_f

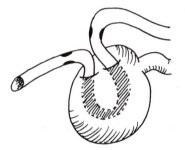 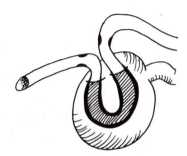

	Normal		**Increase K_f**		**Decrease K_f**	
	Afferent Pressure	Efferent Pressure	Afferent Pressure	Efferent Pressure	Afferent Pressure	Efferent Pressure
	(mm Hg)	(mm Hg)	(mm Hg)	(mm Hg)	(mm Hg)	(mm Hg)
P_c	45	45	45		45	45
π_c	20	35		35	20	
P_{BS}	10		10		10	
π_{BS}	0		0		0	
Net Filtration Pressure (mm Hg)	7.38		7.38		7.38	
K_f (ml/min/mm Hg)	13.5				10	
GFR (ml/min)			111			
RPF	←——→					

Example 1 – Altered K_f: Solution

INCREASED K_f

DECREASED K_f

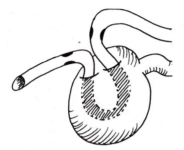
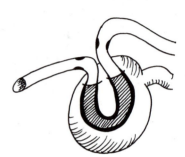

	Normal		Increase K_f		Decrease K_f	
	Afferent Pressure (mm Hg)	Efferent Pressure (mm Hg)	Afferent Pressure (mm Hg)	Efferent Pressure (mm Hg)	Afferent Pressure (mm Hg)	Efferent Pressure (mm Hg)
P_c	45	45	45	45	45	45
π_c	20	35	20	35	20	35
P_{BS}	10		10		10	
π_{BS}	0		0		0	
Net Filtration Pressure (mm Hg)	7.38		7.38		7.38	
K_f (ml/min/mm Hg)	13.5		15		10	
GFR (ml/min)	100		111		74	
RPF	⟷		⟷		⟷	

Example 1 – Altered K_f: Explanation

In this example, and in all examples in this chapter, we assume that P_c does not decrease along the length of the glomerular capillary and that π_c increases until filtration equilibrium is reached. We are also assuming that no protein leaks into Bowman's space (π_{BS} is zero), P_{BS} is ten, and that the increase in π_c along the length of the glomerular capillary follows a natural logarithmic progression.

Net filtration pressure equals the average pressure between P_c and π_c in Figure 1. From the values given for the normal capillary, this value is calculated to be 7.38 mm Hg. To calculate GFR for the normal glomerulus, multiply the net filtration pressure times K_f (7.38 mm Hg × 13.5 ml/min/mm Hg = 100 ml/min).

In the capillary with an increase K_f, you are asked to determine P_c at the efferent end of the glomerular capillary. This value could be deduced logically from one of two methods. 1) You are told to assume that P_c does not decrease along the length of the glomerular capillary; therefore, the afferent P_c and the efferent pressures should both equal 45 mm Hg. 2) Because a point of filtration equilibrium is reached before the end of the glomerular capillary, the force favoring filtration (P_c) and those opposing filtration (π_c and P_{BS}) must be equal. In this example, you know that the force opposing filtration is 45 mm Hg (35 mm Hg + 10 mm Hg).

You are also asked to provide a value for P_c at the afferent end of the glomerular capillary. You can assume that this will be equal to the value given in the example of the normal glomerulus, because changing the permeability of the glomerular capillary (increasing K_f) will not alter this value.

In the example of the capillary with an increase in K_f, you are given GFR and asked to provide a value for K_f. This value can be determined if GFR is divided by the average net filtration pressure (111 ml/mm ÷ 7.38 mm Hg = 15 ml/min/mm Hg).

Increasing K_f should not change resistance along the glomerular capillary; therefore, renal plasma flow should not be changed.

In the final problem of this example, you are asked to provide a value for π_c at the efferent end of the glomerular capillary. To calculate this value, you should remember that unless protein is leaking into Bowman's space, there are two forces that oppose filtration and one force that favors filtration. The sum of these forces must equal zero at the efferent end of the glomerular capillary if filtration equilibrium has been reached. In this chapter, you assume that equilibrium is reached in all examples; therefore, π_c at the efferent end of the glomerular capillary must equal the difference between P_c and P_{BS} (45 mm Hg – 10 mm Hg = 35 mm Hg).

You are asked to calculate GFR. This is accomplished by multiplying the net filtration pressure times K_f (7.38 mm Hg × 10 ml/min/mm Hg = 74 ml/min/mm Hg). Decreasing K_f should not change renal plasma flow.

Example 2 – Altering Afferent π_c: Problem

INCREASING π_c

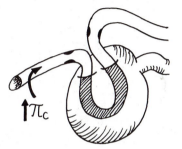

DECREASING π_c

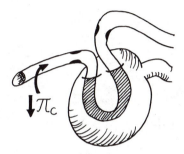

	Normal		Increase Afferent π_c		Decrease Afferent π_c	
	Afferent Pressure (mm Hg)	Efferent Pressure (mm Hg)	Afferent Pressure (mm Hg)	Efferent Pressure (mm Hg)	Afferent Pressure (mm Hg)	Efferent Pressure (mm Hg)
P_c	45	45	45	45	45	45
π_c	20	35	30	35	10	35
P_{BS}	10		10		10	
π_{BS}	0		0		0	
Net Filtration Pressure (mm Hg)	7.38		6.67		7.54	
K_f (ml/min/mm Hg)	13.5		13.5		13.5	
GFR (ml/min)						
RPF	←——→					

Example 2 – Altering Afferent π_c: Solution

INCREASING π_c

DECREASING π_c

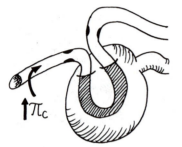

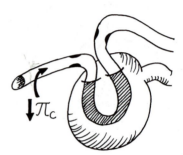

	Normal		Increase Afferent π_c		Decrease Afferent π_c	
	Afferent Pressure (mm Hg)	Efferent Pressure (mm Hg)	Afferent Pressure (mm Hg)	Efferent Pressure (mm Hg)	Afferent Pressure (mm Hg)	Efferent Pressure (mm Hg)
P_c	45	45	45	45	45	45
π_c	20	35	30	35	10	35
P_{BS}	10		10		10	
π_{BS}	0		0		0	
Net Filtration Pressure (mm Hg)	7.38		6.67		7.54	
K_f (ml/min/mm Hg)	13.5		13.5		13.5	
GFR (ml/min)	100		90		102	
RPF	←——→		←——→		←——→	

Example 2 – Altering Afferent π_c: Explanation

The assumptions listed in the previous example and in the introduction apply also to this example. These are as follows: 1) afferent and efferent P_c are equal, 2) π_c increases in a natural logarithmic fashion from the afferent to the efferent end of the glomerular capillary, 3) a point of filtration equilibrium is reached before the end of the glomerular capillary, and 4) no protein leaks across the glomerular capillary; therefore, π_{BS} equals zero)

In the problem illustrating a normal glomerular capillary, you are asked to calculate GFR. This can be accomplished by multiplying the average net filtration pressure times K_f (7.8 mm Hg × 13.5 ml/min/mm Hg = 100 ml/min).

The second problem in this example illustrates an increase in afferent oncotic pressure (π_c) to 30 mm Hg. The other factors considered in Starling's equilibrium equation are assumed to remain constant. Based upon this assumption, it was calculated that the net filtration pressure will decrease to 6.67 mm Hg. In this problem you are asked to calculate GFR. This is accomplished by multiplying the net filtration pressure times K_f (6.67 mm Hg × 13.5 ml/min/mm Hg = 90 ml/min).

Increasing afferent π_c should not affect renal plasma flow.

In the last problem of this example, you are asked to consider the effect of decreasing afferent oncotic pressure (π_c) to 10 mm Hg. If all other factors remain constant, net filtration pressure would increase to 7.54 mm Hg. GFR is calculated by multiplying the net filtration pressure times K_f (7.54 mm Hg × 13.5 ml/min/mm Hg = 102 ml/min).

Decreasing afferent π_c should not change renal plasma flow.

Example 3 – Constriction or Dilation of the Afferent Arteriole: Problem

AFFERENT CONSTRICTION

AFFERENT DILATION

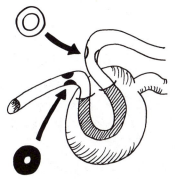
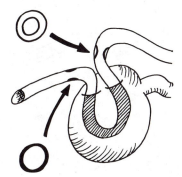

	Normal		Afferent Constriction		Afferent Dilation	
	Afferent Pressure	Efferent Pressure	Afferent Pressure	Efferent Pressure	Afferent Pressure	Efferent Pressure
	(mm Hg)	(mm Hg)	(mm Hg)	(mm Hg)	(mm Hg)	(mm Hg)
P_c	45	45	40		50	
π_c	20	35	20	30	20	40
P_{BS}	10		10		10	
π_{BS}	0		0		0	
Net Filtration Pressure (mm Hg)	7.38		6.21		8.50	
K_f (ml/min/mm Hg)	13.5		13.5		13.5	
GFR (ml/min)						
RPF	← →					

Example 3 – Constriction or Dilation of the Afferent Arteriole: Solution

AFFERENT CONSTRICTION

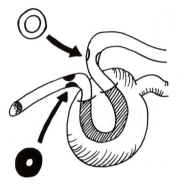

AFFERENT DILATION

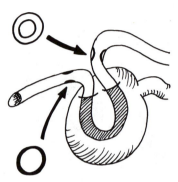

	Normal		Afferent Constriction		Afferent Dilation	
	Afferent Pressure (mm Hg)	Efferent Pressure (mm Hg)	Afferent Pressure (mm Hg)	Efferent Pressure (mm Hg)	Afferent Pressure (mm Hg)	Efferent Pressure (mm Hg)
P_c	45	45	40	40	50	50
π_c	20	35	20	30	20	40
P_{BS}	10		10		10	
π_{BS}	0		0		0	
Net Filtration Pressure (mm Hg)	7.38		6.21		8.50	
K_f (ml/min/mm Hg)	13.5		13.5		13.5	
GFR (ml/min)	100		84		115	
RPF	←→		↓		↑	

Example 3 – Constriction or Dilation of the Afferent Arteriole: Explanation

As indicated in the introduction and in the previous example, several assumptions are made in this chapter regarding glomerular filtration. These include: 1) efferent and afferent capillary hydrostatic pressure are equal, 2) plasma oncotic pressure increases in a natural logarithmic fashion along the length of the glomerular capillary, 3) a point of filtration equilibrium is reached before the end of the glomerular capillary, and 4) the glomerular capillary does not allow the passage of protein; therefore, oncotic pressure in Bowman's space (π_{BS}) is zero.

In the first problem of this example, you are asked to calculate GFR in a normal glomerulus. This is accomplished by multiplying the average net filtration pressure times K_f (7.38 mm Hg × 13.5 ml/min/mm Hg = 100 ml/min).

In the next problem, you are asked to consider the situation that would occur if the afferent arteriole was constricted. Constriction of the afferent arteriole would decrease capillary hydrostatic pressure (P_c). You are told that the afferent hydrostatic pressure is 40 mm Hg. Hydrostatic pressure is assumed to not decrease along the length of the glomerular capillary; therefore, the hydrostatic pressure at the efferent end of the capillary also must be 40 mm Hg. This value could also be determined by an alternative method. Remember that at the point of filtration equilibrium, the forces favoring filtration and those opposing filtration must equal zero. Based upon this, P_c (the force favoring filtration) must equal the sum of the two forces opposing filtration (π_c and P_{BS}).

GFR can be calculated by multiplying the net filtration pressure times K_f (6.21 mm Hg × 13.5 ml/min/mm Hg = 84 ml/min). Constriction of the afferent arteriole will cause a decrease in renal plasma flow.

In the last problem of this example, you are asked to consider the effect of dilating the afferent arteriole. Dilation of the afferent arteriole will increase capillary hydrostatic pressure. You are told that P_c is 50 mm Hg. Based upon these data, the net filtration pressure would increase to 8.50 mm Hg. You are asked to calculate GFR.

This is accomplished by multiplying the net filtration pressure times K_f (8.5 mm Hg × 13.5 ml/min/mm Hg = 115 ml/min).

Dilation of the afferent arteriole will cause renal plasma flow to increase.

Example 4 – Constriction or Dilation of the Efferent Arteriole: Problem

EFFERENT CONSTRICTION

EFFERENT DILATION

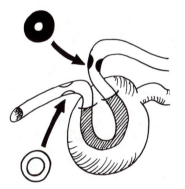
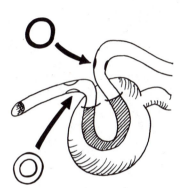

	Normal		Efferent Constriction		Efferent Dilation	
	Afferent Pressure (mm Hg)	Efferent Pressure (mm Hg)	Afferent Pressure (mm Hg)	Efferent Pressure (mm Hg)	Afferent Pressure (mm Hg)	Efferent Pressure (mm Hg)
P_c	45	45	50	50	40	
π_c	20	35	20	40	20	30
P_{BS}	10		10		10	
π_{BS}	0		0		0	
Net Filtration Pressure (mm Hg)	7.38		8.50		6.21	
K_f (ml/min/mm Hg)			13.5		13.5	
GFR (ml/min)	100					
RPF	⟵——⟶					

Example 4 – Constriction or Dilation of the Efferent Arteriole: Solution

EFFERENT CONSTRICTION

EFFERENT DILATION

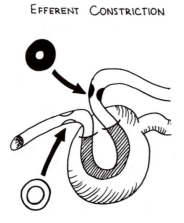
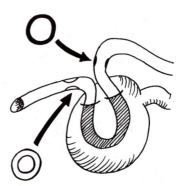

	Normal		Efferent Constriction		Efferent Dilation	
	Afferent Pressure	Efferent Pressure	Afferent Pressure	Efferent Pressure	Afferent Pressure	Efferent Pressure
	(mm Hg)	(mm Hg)	(mm Hg)	(mm Hg)	(mm Hg)	(mm Hg)
P_C	45	45	50	50	40	40
π_C	20	35	20	40	20	30
P_{BS}	10		10		10	
π_{BS}	0		0		0	
Net Filtration Pressure (mm Hg)	7.38		8.50		6.21	
K_f (ml/min/mm Hg)	13.5		13.5		13.5	
GFR (ml/min)	100		115		84	
RPF	⟷		↓		↑	

Example 4 – Constriction or Dilation of the Efferent Arteriole: Explanation

In all examples in this chapter, several assumptions are made. They are: 1) hydrostatic pressure does not decrease along the length of the glomerular capillary, 2) oncotic pressure increases in a logarithmic fashion from the afferent to the efferent end of the glomerular capillary, 3) a point of filtration equilibrium is reached before the end of the glomerular capillary, and 4) the glomerular capillary is impermeable to protein; therefore, π_c is zero.

Based upon the data given for the normal capillary, it was calculated that the average filtration pressure is 7.38 mm Hg. You are asked to calculate K_f in this problem. This is accomplished by dividing GFR by the average net filtration pressure (100 ml/min ÷ 7.38 mm Hg = 13.5 ml/min/mm Hg).

In the second problem of this example, you are asked to consider the situation that would exist if the efferent arteriole was constricted. You are told that this will increase hydrostatic pressure in the glomerular capillary to 50 mm Hg. Based upon these data, the net filtration pressure in the glomerular capillary increases to 8.5 mm Hg. GFR is calculated by multiplying the average net filtration pressure times K_f (8.5 mm Hg × 13.5 ml/min/mm Hg = 115 ml/min).

Constriction of the efferent arteriole would cause renal plasma flow to decrease.

In the last problem of this example, you are asked to consider the effects that are produced by dilation of the efferent arteriole. You are told that in this problem P_c would be decreased to 40 mm Hg. Based upon these data, the net filtration pressure would be 6.21 mm Hg. GFR is calculated by multiplying the net filtration pressure times K_f (6.21 mm Hg × 13.5 ml/min/mm Hg = 84 ml/min).

Dilation of the efferent arteriole will cause renal plasma flow to increase.

Summary

Starling's noteworthy experiments conducted at the turn of the century helped resolve the debate between Ludwig and Bowman. Unfortunately, many other issues remain to be resolved. Several of the assumptions in this chapter are simplifications of the actual events because our understanding of these events is lacking. For example, we assume that hydrostatic pressure does not decrease along the length of the glomerular capillary; however, some decrease in pressure undoubtedly occurs.

Oncotic pressure is assumed to increase in a natural logarithmic fashion as the fluid moves along the length of the glomerular capillary. Although many biological events follow a natural logarithmic progression, we are uncertain if the change in capillary oncotic pressure along the glomerulus is one such event. It is generally accepted that the rate of change is more rapid in the earlier sections of the capillary, but the rate at which this change occurs has not been determined.

We also assumed, that a point of filtration equilibrium, or balance between the forces favoring and opposing filtration, is reached before the end of the glomerular capillary. The equation we used to calculated the average net filtration pressure assumed that the site along the glomerular capillary where filtration equilibrium was reached remained constant. Most likely, the site along the length of the glomerular capillary where filtration equilibrium occurs changes with alterations in renal plasma flow, plasma oncotic pressure, and capillary hydrostatic pressure change. Once again, our knowledge in this area is lacking.

The equation we used to calculate net filtration pressure did not consider several other variables that may be important in the calculation of this value. For example, flow rate along the glomerular capillary may play an important role in determining the change in plasma oncotic pressure.

Starling's work helped solve one point of disagreement, but posed many new questions that remain unresolved. Solutions to these new questions are more difficult to address and have eluded scientists for many years. The following statements represent our knowledge of the glomerular filtration as scientists currently understand the mechanisms involved in this process.

Arteriole constriction—Constricting either the afferent or efferent arteriole will decrease renal plasma flow because the two arterioles are in series and their resistance is additive. If the afferent arteriole is constricted, pressure in the glomerular capillary will decrease, which will decrease GFR. If the efferent arteriole is constricted, pressure in the glomerular capillary will increase and GFR will increase.

Arteriole dilation—Dilation of either the afferent or efferent arteriole will increase renal plasma flow because the arterioles are in series and the resistance is additive. Dilation of the afferent arteriole will increase pressure in the glomerular capillary and will increase GFR. Dilation of the efferent arteriole will decrease glomerular hydrostatic pressure and will decrease GFR.

Altering afferent oncotic pressure—Increasing or decreasing the oncotic pressure of the plasma entering the glomerulus will alter glomerular filtration rate. Increasing afferent plasma oncotic pressure will result in a decreased net filtration pressure and will decrease GFR. Decreasing afferent plasma oncotic pressure will increase net filtration pressure and increase GFR.

Altering capillary permeability—Altering capillary permeability will alter GFR. By using the Starling equilibrium equation you can see that increasing capillary permeability (K_f) will increase GFR, whereas decreasing capillary permeability will decrease GFR. This change in GFR will occur with no change in the forces that favor or oppose the filtration process.

Many pathological conditions that were not covered in this chapter can significantly alter glomerular filtration. Pathological conditions that affect plasma proteins will alter plasma oncotic pressure and alter glomerular filtration rate. The permeability of the glomerular capillary is altered by a number of disease processes that thicken the filtration barrier. Many of these diseases cause the deposition of immuno-complexes on the basement membrane. Alterations in glomerular hydrostatic pressure can occur from vascular diseases or clots that can form in the renal artery. Such changes can decrease renal blood flow to a point that will stop glomerular filtration. Consideration of these pathological problems are beyond the scope of this chapter, but can be reviewed in nephrology, pathology, or most general internal medicine texts.

INULIN EXCRETION

Introduction

Inulin is a polysaccharide found in Jerusalem artichokes. It has a molecular weight of approximately 5,000 Daltons and is not secreted or reabsorbed by the renal tubules. These characteristics give the compound several properties that make it useful to the renal physiologist. First, the relatively low molecular weight (and lack of molecular charge) ensures it is freely filtered and appears in Bowman's space at a concentration equal to its concentration in the plasma flowing through the glomerular capillary. Second, it is similar in molecular structure to compounds the body uses as nutrients. Thus, the kidney excretes the compound by filtration only, instead of secreting it as it would a toxic compound. Third, inulin cannot be metabolized by the body; therefore, the kidney does not reabsorb this compound as it would, for example, glucose. Because inulin is not reabsorbed, the amount/min filtered into Bowman's space is equal to the amount/min excreted into the urine. The concentration of inulin in the urine is greater than the concentration in the glomerular filtrate because water is reabsorbed along the length of the tubule.

Other compounds have characteristics that are similar to inulin; however, none have the same properties that make inulin so useful to the renal physiologist. For example, creatinine is freely filtered like inulin, but it is also secreted in small amounts by the human kidney. Clinicians frequently use creatinine clearance instead of inulin to calculate GFR (glomerular filtration rate) in patients. The slight tubular secretion of creatinine causes a small error in the calculation but other characteristics make it quite useful in the clinical setting. For example, inulin has to be injected or infused into the patient at a given rate while clearance is being measured, whereas creatinine is an endogenously occurring compound that is normally maintained at a constant rate.

The following examples are designed to stimulate your problem solving skills and help you develop a logical understanding of how inulin and similar compounds are handled by the renal tubules. Try to solve for all the missing spaces on the chart in example 1 by using the formulae you are given in the definitions. Remember you may have to perform some intermediate steps (conversions) to get the values necessary for the calculations.

It is not enough to check your answers quickly to the given solutions. Active learning requires that you review the explanation carefully to ensure you arrived at the answers using the correct formulae. A firm understanding of the logic used in arriving at the solution is necessary before you move on to the next example.

Objectives

- Explain why the concentration of a freely filtered compound is equal in the afferent arteriole, Bowman's space, and efferent arteriole.

- Explain how renal plasma flow can be calculated using the Fick equation.

- Define clearance and explain how the clearance equation is used to calculate this volume.

- Explain why the clearance of inulin is equal to GFR.

- Explain the concept of G-T balance.

- Explain why the TF/P ratio for inulin is important in determining how other compounds are handled by the renal tubules.

- Graph the TF/P ratio for inulin in each section of the renal tubule.

- Define and explain the concept of mass balance.

- Define extraction ratio and explain how it is calculated.

- Explain why the extraction ratio for inulin is equal to filtration fraction.

- Explain how filtration fraction is calculated.

- Calculate the various values requested in each example and explain how each value is determined.

- Explain why the clearance of inulin is not affected by its plasma concentration.

- Explain why the clearance of creatinine is often used to estimate GFR.

- Define filtered load and show how it is calculated.

Example 1: Problem

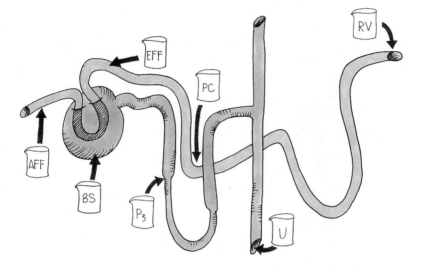

Site	Amount/min (mg / min)	Flow Rate (ml / min)	Concentration (mg / ml)	TF/P ratio
AFF	**500**	**500**		
BS				
EFF				
P3				
PC				
RV				
U	**100**	**1**		

G-T balance _____ $^2/_3$ _____

Clearance _____

RPF _____

Extraction ratio _____

Filtration fraction _____

Tm _____

Example 1: Solution

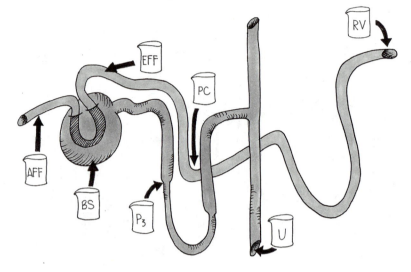

Site	Amount/min (mg / min)	Flow Rate (ml / min)	Concentration (mg / ml)	TF/P ratio
AFF	**500**	**500**	1	
BS	100	100	1	1
EFF	400	400	1	
P3	100	33	3	3
PC	400	467		
RV	400	499	0.8	
U	**100**	**1**	100	100

G-T balance _____ 2/3 _____

Clearance _____ 100 _____

RPF _____ 500 _____

Extraction ratio _____ 0.20 _____

Filtration fraction _____ 0.20 _____

Tm _____ N/A _____

Example 1: Explanation

The amount/min of inulin and the flow rate of plasma at site AFF are given. From these data, the concentration of inulin at site AFF is 1 mg/ml.

$$\text{Concentration } (P_{in}) = \frac{\text{Amount/min}}{\text{Flow Rate}} = \frac{500 \text{ mg/min}}{500 \text{ ml/min}} = 1 \text{ mg /ml}$$

Inulin is neither secreted nor reabsorbed. Therefore, the amount/min of inulin excreted at site U (given) must be equal to the amount/min of inulin at site BS, or 100 mg/min. The volume appearing at site BS per minute is the GFR. GFR is equal to the amount/min of inulin excreted divided by the concentration of inulin in the afferent arteriole.

$$\text{GFR} = \text{Flow Rate at site BS} = \frac{100 \text{ mg/min}}{1 \text{mg/ml}} = 100 \text{ ml/min}$$

The concentration of inulin at sites AFF, BS, and EFF is always equal if the compound is freely filtered. Under these conditions, the TF/P ratio at site BS always equals one.

The amount/min of inulin found at site EFF must equal the amount/min at site AFF minus the amount/min at site BS if mass balance is to be maintained. Similarly, the flow rate at site EFF must equal the flow rate at site AFF minus the flow rate at site BS.

You calculated that the flow rate at site BS (GFR) is 100 ml/min. The G-T balance is given as two-thirds, which means that two-thirds of the volume filtered per minute is reabsorbed in the proximal tubule; therefore, 33 ml/min must remain at the end of the proximal tubule.

$$\text{Flow Rate at P3} = \text{GFR} \times (1 - \text{G-T Balance})$$
$$= 100 \text{ ml/min} \times 1/3 = 33 \text{ ml/min}$$

None of the filtered inulin is reabsorbed in the proximal tubule and no inulin is secreted. Thus, the amount/min of inulin appearing at the end of the proximal tubule (site P3) must equal the amount/min filtered (site BS). The TF/P ratio for inulin at site P3 reflects the ratio of filtered water that is reabsorbed in the proximal tubule (G-T balance). For example, a G-T balance of two-thirds results in a TF/P_{in} ratio of three at the end of the proximal tubule. This is calculated by dividing the concentration at site P3 by the concentration at site AFF.

$$TF/P \text{ ratio at site P3} = \frac{\text{Concentration at P3}}{\text{Concentration at AFF}} = \frac{3 \text{ mg/ml}}{1 \text{ mg/ml}} = 3$$

The flow rate of plasma at site PC is equal to the flow rate at site EFF plus the volume per minute that is reabsorbed in the proximal tubule. Because 100 ml/min of plasma is filtered into Bowman's space and two-thirds of that is reabsorbed, 67 ml/min are added to the 400 ml/min at site EFF to give a flow rate of 467 ml/min at site PC.

$$\text{Flow Rate at PC} = \text{Flow Rate at EFF} + (\text{GFR} \times \text{G-T Balance})$$
$$= 400 + 67 = 467 \text{ ml/min.}$$

Inulin is not transported by the renal tubule; therefore, the amount/min found at site EFF must equal the amount/min found at site PC.

Remember that to maintain mass balance, the amount/min at site P3 plus the amount/min at site PC must equal the amount/min at site AFF. This is also true for the flow rate at these sites. Also to maintain mass balance, the flow rate of plasma found at site RV must equal the flow rate entering the kidney at site AFF minus the urine flow rate. Similarly, the amount/min of inulin at site RV must equal the amount/min entering the kidney minus the amount/min excreted in the urine.

The urine flow rate and the amount/min of inulin appearing at site U per minute are given. (To maintain mass balance, the flow rate at site U plus the flow rate at site RV must equal the flow rate at site AFF, and the amount/min at site U plus site RV must equal the amount/min at site AFF). The concentration of inulin is calculated by dividing the amount/min by the flow rate.

$$\text{Concentration at U} = \frac{\text{Amount/min at U}}{\text{Flow Rate at U}} = \frac{100 \text{ mg/min}}{1 \text{ ml/min}} = 100 \text{ mg/ml}$$

The TF/P ratio at site U is equal to this concentration divided by the concentration of inulin at site AFF.

$$\text{TF}/\text{P} \text{ ratio at U} = \frac{\text{Concentration at U}}{\text{Concentration at AFF}} = \frac{100 \text{ mg}/\text{ml}}{1 \text{ mg}/\text{ml}} = 100$$

The concentration at site RV is equal to the amount/min at site RV divided by the flow rate at site RV (400 mg/min ÷ 499 ml/min = 0.8 mg/ml).

Clearance is calculated by dividing the amount/min of inulin excreted (site U) by the plasma concentration (site AFF). Remember that the clearance of inulin is equal to GFR. GFR is also equal to the flow rate at site BS, which you have already calculated.

$$C_{in} = GFR = \frac{100 \text{ mg}/\text{min}}{1\text{mg}/\text{ml}} = 100 \text{ ml}/\text{min}$$

RPF can be calculated by several methods. The commonly used method divides the amount/min of inulin excreted (site BS) by the difference between the concentration in the renal artery (site AFF) and the concentration in the renal vein (site RV).

$$RPF = \frac{Qe}{Pa_x - Pv_x} = \frac{100}{1 - 0.8} = 500 \text{ ml}/\text{min}$$

This calculated RPF flow rate equals the flow rate at site AFF.

The extraction ratio equals the difference between the concentration in the renal artery (site AFF) and the concentration in the renal vein (site RV) divided by the concentration in the renal artery.

$$E_x = \frac{Pa_x - Pv_x}{Pa_x} = \frac{1 \text{ mg}/\text{ml} - 0.8 \text{ mg}/\text{ml}}{1 \text{ mg}/\text{ml}} = 0.20$$

(Remember that the extraction ratio for inulin is equal to the filtration fraction).

The filtration fraction is equal to GFR divided by renal plasma flow.

$$FF = \frac{100 \text{ ml}/\text{min}}{500 \text{ ml}/\text{min}} = 0.2$$

Example 2: Problem

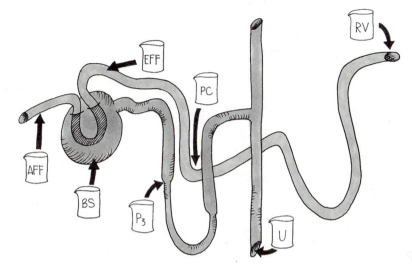

Site	Amount/min (mg / min)	Flow Rate (ml / min)	Concentration (mg / ml)	TF/P ratio
AFF			2	░░░
BS		50		
EFF		450		░░░
P3				
PC			░░░	░░░
RV			░░░	░░░
U	100	2		

G-T balance _____ ²/₃ _____

Clearance _____

RPF _____

Extraction ratio _____

Filtration fraction _____

Tm _____

Example 2: Solution

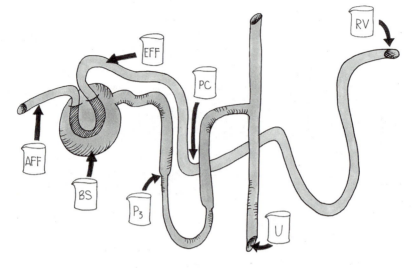

Site	Amount/min (mg / min)	Flow Rate (ml / min)	Concentration (mg / ml)	TF/P ratio
AFF	1000	500	**2**	
BS	100	**50**	2	1
EFF	900	**450**	2	
P3	100	16.5	6	3
PC	900	483.5		
RV	900	498	1.8	
U	**100**	**2**	50	25

G-T balance	2/3
Clearance	50
RPF	500
Extraction ratio	0.1
Filtration fraction	0.1
Tm	N/A

Example 2: Explanation

To solve this example, you first need to remember that the concentration of a freely filtered compound is the same at sites AFF, BS, and EFF. For this example that concentration is given as 2 mg/ml. If you multiply this concentration by the flow rate at sites BS and EFF, you can calculate that the amount/min of inulin appearing in Bowman's space (site BS) is 100 mg/min and the amount/min appearing in the efferent arteriole is 900 mg/min. From example 1, you learned that the TF/P ratio at site BS always equals one for inulin or any freely filtered compound.

The amount/min at site AFF must equal the amount/min at site BS plus the amount/min at site EFF. Using this logic, you can determine that the amount/min entering the afferent arteriole (site AFF) is 1000 mg/min. The flow rate at site AFF is calculated by adding the flow rates at site BS and site EFF.

Inulin is neither secreted nor reabsorbed; therefore, the 100 mg/min of inulin that entered Bowman's space (site BS) appear at site P3 and at site U. Based on this same principle, 900 mg/min of inulin appear at site PC and at site RV.

The G-T balance is given as two-thirds. Using this value you can calculate that the rate of flow at the end of the proximal tubule is 16.5 ml/min. The concentration at site P3 is equal to the amount/min at site P3 divided by the flow rate at site P3. The TF/P ratio at site P3 is three (review example 1).

The volume per minute that is reabsorbed from the proximal tubule (33.5 ml/min) is returned to the peritubular capillary. This is added to the flow rate in the efferent arteriole (given as 450 ml/min) so that the flow rate reaching site PC is 483.5 ml/min. (Review example 1 if you could not calculate these values.)

The urine flow rate is given as 2 ml/min. The flow rate in the renal vein must be the difference between the 500 ml/min that enters the kidney and the 2 ml/min that are excreted as urine.

The concentration at site RV is equal to the amount/min at site RV divided by the flow rate at site RV. The concentration at site U is calculated by dividing the amount/min of inulin at site U by the flow rate appearing at that site . The TF/P ratio at site U is calculated by dividing the concentration at site U by the concentration at site AFF.

In this example the flow rate at site BS is also equal to the clearance. This same flow rate can be calculated by dividing the amount of the compound excreted per minute (amount/min at site U) by the plasma concentration (concentration at site AFF).

Renal plasma flow can be calculated using several methods. Using our standard equation, RPF is calculated by dividing the amount of the compound excreted per minute by the difference in concentration between site AFF and site RV. Or, renal plasma flow can be calculated by adding the flow rate appearing at site BS and at site EFF. Remember that mass balance must be maintained between these three sites.

The extraction ratio is determined using the standard equation for this value. The difference between the concentration at site AFF and site RV is divided by the concentration at site AFF.

Filtration fraction is equal to GFR divided by RPF. From example 1 you know that the extraction ratio for inulin and the filtration fraction are always equal.

Example 3: Problem

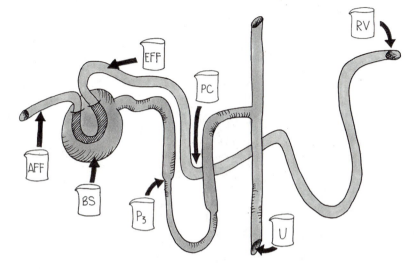

Site	Amount/min (mg / min)	Flow Rate (ml / min)	Concentration (mg / ml)	TF/P ratio
AFF				
BS		100		
EFF			1.5	
P3		25		
PC				
RV		599		
U				

G-T balance _____

Clearance _____

RPF _____ **600 ml/min**

Extraction ratio _____

Filtration fraction _____

Tm _____

Example 3: Solution

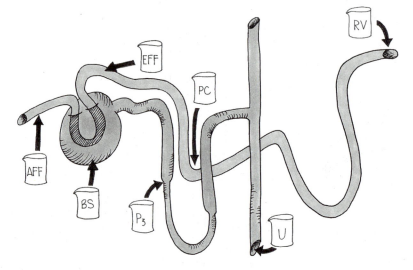

Site	Amount/min (mg / min)	Flow Rate (ml / min)	Concentration (mg / ml)	TF/P ratio
AFF	900	600	1.5	
BS	150	**100**	1.5	1
EFF	750	500	**1.5**	
P3	150	**25**	6	4
PC	750	575		
RV	750	**599**	1.25	
U	150	1	150	100

G-T balance _____ $^3/_4$ _____

Clearance _____ 100 _____

RPF _____ **600 ml/min** _____

Extraction ratio _____ 0.167 _____

Filtration fraction _____ 0.167 _____

Tm _____ N/A _____

Example 3: Explanation

The concentration of inulin (or any freely filtered compound) is the same at sites AFF, BS, and EFF. Renal plasma flow (the flow rate appearing at site AFF) is given as 600 ml/min. With this data you can determine that the amount/min of the compound appearing at site AFF is 900 mg/min and the amount/min of the compound appearing at site BS is 150 mg/min. Subtract the amount/min at site BS from the amount/min at site AFF to get the amount/min at site EFF. Using the same logic, you can calculate the flow rate appearing at site EFF.

All of the filtered inulin (site BS) remains in the renal tubule and appears in the urine. Therefore, the amount/min of inulin appearing at site BS is also found at site P3 and at site U. To maintain mass balance, the remainder of the 900 mg/min that entered the kidney must appear at site PC and site RV (900 mg/min – 150 mg/min = 750 mg/min).

From previous examples you know that the TF/P ratio at BS always equals one for inulin or any other freely filtered compound. The concentration of inulin at site P3 equals the amount/min at site P3 divided by the flow rate at site P3. The TF/P ratio at site P3 is affected by the percentage of filtered water that is reabsorbed in the proximal tubule. In this example, the TF/P ratio at site P3 is four because three-fourths of the filtered water is reabsorbed in the proximal tubule.

You are given that 25 ml/min appear at site P3. This means that of the 100 ml/min filtered into Bowman's space at site BS, 25 ml/min are reabsorbed into the peritubular capillary. This means that 575 ml/min appear at site PC.

You are given that 599 ml/min appear at site RV. To maintain mass balance, the urine flow rate must be the difference between this flow rate and the flow rate that originally entered the afferent arteriole (600 ml/min – 1 ml/min = 599 ml/min).

G-T balance is equal to the volume of fluid reabsorbed in the proximal tubule divided by GFR. Of the 100 ml/min that are filtered into Bowman's space, 25 ml/min reached the end of the proximal tubule; therefore, 75 ml/min are reabsorbed. This is used to calculate a G-T balance of three-fourths.

$$G - T \text{ Balance} = \frac{GFR - \text{Flow Rate at P3}}{GFR}$$

$$= \frac{100 \text{ ml/min} - 25 \text{ ml/min}}{100 \text{ ml/min}} = \frac{75 \text{ ml/min}}{100 \text{ ml/min}} = \frac{3}{4}$$

Clearance is equal to the amount excreted per minute divided by the plasma concentration at site AFF.

Renal plasma flow is given. RPF is equal to the flow rate at site AFF and was used earlier in your calculations.

The extraction ratio is equal to the difference between the concentration in the afferent arteriole (site AFF) and the concentration in the renal vein (site RV) divided by the concentration in the afferent arteriole.

Filtration fraction is that fraction of renal plasma flow that appears in Bowman's space as glomerular filtrate. This is calculated by dividing the flow rate at site BS by the flow rate at site AFF or GFR divided by RPF.

Example 4: Problem

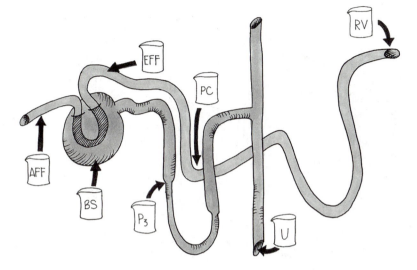

Site	Amount/min (mg / min)	Flow Rate (ml / min)	Concentration (mg / ml)	TF/P ratio
AFF				
BS				
EFF			1	
P3				
PC				
RV				
U		2		50

G-T balance _____ 2/3 _____

Clearance _____

RPF _____

Extraction ratio _____

Filtration fraction ___ **0.20** _____

Tm _____

Example 4: Solution

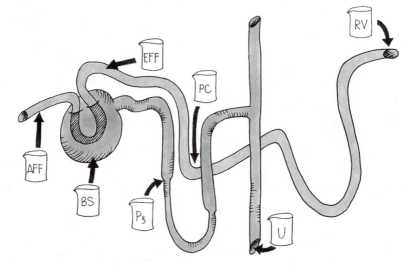

Site	Amount/min (mg / min)	Flow Rate (ml / min)	Concentration (mg / ml)	TF/P ratio
AFF	500	500	1	
BS	100	100	1	1
EFF	400	400	1	
P3	100	33	3	3
PC	400	467		
RV	400	498	0.8	
U	100	**2**	50	**50**

G-T balance _____ 2/3 _____

Clearance _____ 100 _____

RPF _____ 500 _____

Extraction ratio _____ 0.20 _____

Filtration fraction ___ 0.20 _____

Tm _____ N/A _____

Example 4: Explanation

The concentration at site EFF is given and you know that the concentration of inulin at sites AFF, BS, and EFF is always equal. You are given that the TF/P ratio for inulin at site U is 50. With this data you can calculate that the concentration at site U must be 50 mg/min.

By knowing the flow rate and concentration at site U, you can determine the amount of inulin appearing in the urine per minute (site U) to be 100 mg/min. Because inulin is neither secreted nor reabsorbed, the amount/min of inulin appearing in the urine must equal the amount/min of inulin that is filtered in Bowman's space (site BS) and the amount/min appearing at the end of the proximal tubule (site P3).

Filtration fraction is equal to glomerular filtration rate divided by renal plasma flow. The filtration fraction is given as 0.2. You can use this value and the GFR to calculate that RPF (at site AFF) is 500 ml/min. To maintain mass balance, the flow rate at site EFF must equal the difference between the flow rates appearing at sites AFF and BS.

Now that you know the flow rates at sites AFF, BS, and EFF and the concentration at each of those sites, you can determine the amount/min appearing at each site by multiplying the appropriate flow rate by the concentration.

The G-T balance is given as two-thirds. Using this value, you can calculate the flow rate at site P3 to be 33 ml/min and the flow rate appearing at site PC to be 467 ml/min.

The amount/min of inulin appearing in Bowman's space is equal to the amount/min appearing at each site along the rest of the renal tubule. Based on this, you can assume that the amount/min of inulin at site P3 and the amount/min of inulin at site U are equal to 100 mg/min. Using this same logic, the amount/min of inulin appearing at site EFF must also equal the amount/min of inulin appearing at site PC and at site RV.

The flow rate of urine is given as 2 ml/min. To maintain mass balance the remainder of the 500 ml/min that entered the afferent arteriole (site AFF) must appear in the renal vein (site RV).

The concentration of inulin in the renal vein is equal to the flow rate in the renal vein divided into the amount/min of inulin appearing there or 0.8 mg/ml.

Clearance is calculated by dividing the amount/min of inulin excreted by the plasma concentration at site AFF.

Renal plasma flow initially had to be calculated from the data that the filtration fraction is 0.20 and that GFR is calculated to be 100 ml/min. After the chart has been completed, you can see that renal plasma flow is also equal to the amount of the compound excreted per minute divided by the difference in concentration between site AFF and site RV.

The extraction ratio is equal to the difference between the concentration at site AFF and site RV divided by the concentration at site AFF.

Example 5: Problem

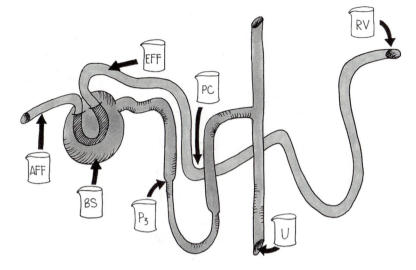

Site	Amount/min (mg / min)	Flow Rate (ml / min)	Concentration (mg / ml)	TF/P ratio
AFF		**500**		
BS			**0.5**	
EFF				
P3				
PC				
RV				
U		**1**	**50**	

G-T balance _____ ³/₄ _____

Clearance _____

RPF _____

Extraction ratio _____

Filtration fraction _____

Tm _____

55

Example 5: Solution

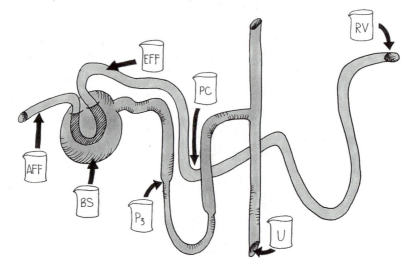

Site	Amount/min (mg / min)	Flow Rate (ml / min)	Concentration (mg / ml)	TF/P ratio
AFF	250	**500**	0.5	
BS	50	100	**0.5**	1
EFF	200	400	0.5	
P3	50	25	2	4
PC	200	475		
RV	200	499	0.4	
U	50	**1**	**50**	100

G-T balance ___ 3/4 ___

Clearance ___ 100 ___

RPF ___ 500 ___

Extraction ratio ___ 0.2 ___

Filtration fraction ___ 0.2 ___

Tm ___ N/A ___

Example 5: Explanation

The plasma concentration of inulin is the same at sites AFF, BS, and EFF. You also know that the TF/P ratio at site BS for such a compound is one. The renal plasma flow at site AFF is given as 500 ml/min. The amount/min of inulin appearing at site AFF is calculated by multiplying the concentration by the flow rate (250 mg/min). You are also given that the urine flow rate is 1 ml/min and the concentration of the urine is 50 mg/ml. With this information you can determine that the amount excreted per minute is 50 mg/min. All of the inulin appearing in the urine must be filtered in Bowman's space because inulin is neither excreted nor reabsorbed. Because of this, the amount/min appearing at site BS must also equal 50 mg/min. By knowing the amount appearing at site BS per minute and the concentration at site BS, you can determine that the flow rate at site BS (GFR) is 100 ml/min. To maintain mass balance, the flow rate at site EFF must be the difference between the flow rate at site AFF and site BS. Likewise, the amount/min at site EFF is the difference between the amount/min appearing at sites AFF and BS.

Because no inulin is reabsorbed along the length of the renal tubule, the amount/min appearing at site P3 must equal the amount/min at site BS (and at site U). Likewise, the amount/min appearing in the peritubular capillary at site EFF must also equal the amount/min appearing at sites PC and RV.

The G-T balance is given as three-fourths, which means that three-fourths of GFR is reabsorbed from the proximal tubule leaving one-fourth of GFR to appear at site P3. Based on this, you can determine that the flow rate at site P3 is 25 ml/min and the flow rate at site PC is 475 ml/min.

The concentration of inulin at site P3 equals the amount/min at site P3 divided by the flow rate at site P3. The TF/P ratio at site P3 is the concentration at this site divided by the concentration at site AFF.

Urine flow rate is given as 1 ml/min. If mass balance is maintained, the flow rate in the renal vein (site RV) must be 499 ml/min. The concentration at site RV is determined by dividing the flow rate at site RV into the amount/min at site RV (0.4 mg/ml).

The TF/P ratio at site U is equal to the concentration of inulin at site U (50 mg/ml) divided by concentration at site AFF (0.5 mg/ml).

The G-T balance is given as three-fourths.

The clearance value was calculated as indicated above; however, you can see that it is also equal to the amount of compound excreted per minute divided by the plasma concentration.

Renal plasma flow is given (flow rate at site AFF). It is also equal to the amount excreted per minute divided by the difference between the concentration in the afferent arteriole and the concentration in the renal vein.

Extraction ratio is the difference between the concentration at site AFF and site RV divided by the concentration at site AFF.

Filtration fraction is equal to glomerular filtration rate divided by renal plasma flow.

Summary

The initial use of inulin as a marker for the determination of glomerular filtration rate was both a brilliant calculation and good fortune. The characteristics of the compound that were mentioned in the introduction to this section have allowed renal physiologists to use inulin to calculate glomerular filtration rate using a simple derivation of the original Fick equation. The Fick equation is also used to measure cardiac output and to estimate renal plasma flow.

amount/min filtered = amount/min excreted

The equation can be explained as follows: the amount/min of inulin filtered is equal to the amount/min of inulin excreted (in the bucket diagrams, the amount/min at site BS is equal to the amount/min at site U) because inulin is neither secreted into the renal tubules nor reabsorbed from them. Further, we know that the amount/min filtered is equal to the flow rate of filtrate formed, multiplied by the concentration of inulin in the filtrate. In the bucket diagrams, the amount/min at site BS (Bowman's space) is equal to the flow rate appearing there times the concentration of inulin appearing in that space. Although it is impossible to measure the concentration of inulin in Bowman's space, we know that this concentration is equal to the plasma concentration because inulin is freely filtered.

Next, we need to determine the amount of inulin excreted per minute. This can be determined by collecting the urine for a known period of time so that the flow rate can be calculated and by measuring the concentration of inulin in this sample. In the bucket diagrams, the amount/min of inulin excreted in the urine (site U) is equal to the urine flow rate multiplied by the concentration of inulin in the urine.

As previously stated, inulin is neither secreted nor reabsorbed by the renal tubules. If this is true, the amount/min of inulin filtered must equal the amount/min of inulin excreted. Based on this logic, the following applies:

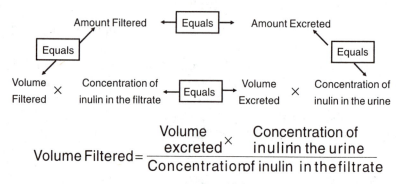

$$\text{Volume Filtered} = \frac{\text{Volume excreted} \times \text{Concentration of inulin in the urine}}{\text{Concentration of inulin in the filtrate}}$$

We know that inulin is freely filtered so that the concentration in the glomerular filtrate is equal to the concentration in the glomerular capillary. Because of this, we can substitute the plasma concentration of inulin for the glomerular concentration of inulin. When this is done, we have the commonly used equation.

$$\text{GFR} = \frac{U_{in}\dot{V}}{P_{in}}$$

where:

U_{in} = Urine concentration of inulin (mg/min)

$\dot{V}$ = Urine flow rate (ml/min)

P_{in} = Plasma concentration of inulin

Initial testing of a patient to determine if they have renal failure may, in part, rely on a simple plasma creatinine and urea level. Most of the creatinine and urea that are excreted enter the renal tubule by the process of filtration. Therefore, if the filtration process is impaired, the plasma concentration of creatinine and urea would be expected to increase.

If a patient is found to have an elevated creatinine and urea concentrations (usually reported as BUN—Blood Urea Nitrogen level), then additional testing to estimate GFR may be warranted. In the clinical setting, creatinine rather than inulin is used to calculate GFR. First, creatinine is an endogenous compound and does not have to be injected into the patient. Second, creatinine is handled in a manner similar to inulin. The small amount of creatinine that is secreted usually is considered insignificant in the clinical setting and produces only a small overestimation of GFR. Third, the plasma concentration of creatinine usually is stable across a 24-hour period, even in a patient with renal failure. Therefore, the blood sample used to determine the plasma concentration does not have to be collected at a specific time during the 24-hour period. Creatinine clearance is measured by collecting the patient's urine for a 24-hour period and determining the concentration of creatinine in this urine sample. A blood sample drawn during or at the end of the 24-hour period is used to determine the plasma concentration. With these values the physician can estimate GFR using the same equation we used above to calculate GFR with inulin; however, the 24-hour creatinine clearance is slightly higher than the value determined with inulin because some creatinine is secreted by the proximal tubule. This small amount usually is considered insignificant and is offset by the relative ease with which the 24-hour creatinine clearance can be calculated compared to the problems encountered in performing the same calculation with inulin.

In the early 1900s, the concept of clearance was introduced by Thomas Addis. Clearance is defined as the volume of plasma that originally contained the amount of a compound excreted per minute. The equation used to calculate this volume is the same equation we used to calculate glomerular filtration rate. The clearance of any compound can be calculated with this equation; however, only the clearance of inulin (or a compound handled by the kidney in a similar fashion) will provide us with the glomerular filtration rate. A compound such as PAH that is both filtered and secreted by the kidney will have a clearance higher than that of inulin, whereas a compound such as glucose that is filtered but reabsorbed will have a clearance value less than that of inulin. This concept is discussed in more detail in later sections.

Renal plasma flow can be calculated using the Fick equation. The bucket diagrams demonstrate how this can be done using inulin. The Fick equation allows us to calculate the flow rate of plasma that enters the kidney via the afferent arteriole. This is accomplished by dividing the amount/min of the compound excreted by the difference between the concentration in the afferent arteriole (site AFF in the bucket diagrams) and the concentration in the renal vein (site RV in the bucket diagrams). The examples in this section use inulin as the compound being measured; however, any freely filtered compound that is not totally reabsorbed by the kidney will suffice.

$$RPF = \frac{U_{in}\dot{V}}{Pa_{in} - Pv_{in}}$$

where:

U_{in}	=	Urine concentration on inulin (mg/ml)
$\dot{V}$	=	Urine flow rate (ml/min)
Pa_{in}	=	Concentration of inulin in the afferent arteriole (mg/ml)
Pv_{in}	=	Concentration of inulin in the renal vein (mg/ml)

This equation overestimates renal plasma flow to a slight extent because the flow rate of urine that is formed per minute causes the concentration in the renal vein to be higher. An explanation of this is found in the Corrections Section.

For each of the inulin examples that were given, the extraction ratio of inulin is always equal to the filtration fraction. The mathematical explanation for this is as follows:

$$FF = \frac{GFR}{RPF}$$

If we write this equation to show the actual parameters involved, we have:

$$FF = \frac{\dfrac{U_{in}\dot{V}}{P_{in}}}{\dfrac{U_{in}\dot{V}}{Pa_{in} - Pv_{in}}}$$

Where:

U_{in}	=	Urine concentration of inulin
$\dot{V}$	=	Urine flow rate
Pa_{in}	=	Renal arterial concentration of inulin
Pv_{in}	=	Renal vein concentration of inulin
P_{in}	=	Concentration of inulin in the general venous concentration (this is equal to Pa in)

If we invert the right hand side of the equation and multiply:

$$FF = \frac{U_{in}\dot{V}}{P_{in}} \times \frac{Pa_{in} - Pv_{in}}{U_{in}\dot{V}}$$

After simplification, we have:

$$FF = \frac{Pa_{in} - Pv_{in}}{P_{in}}$$

This equation is also used to calculate the extraction ratio for inulin. This result is possible only with a compound such as inulin that is freely filtered in the glomerulus and is not secreted or reabsorbed in the tubules. If a compound is transported across the renal tubule, the clearance equation will not give us a measure of glomerular filtration rate, therefore invalidating the assumptions of this calculation.

Several graphs may help to explain the concepts we have covered regarding inulin excretion. If the amount/min of inulin appearing at various sites along the renal tubule is plotted (Figure 3), we find that it remains a constant value throughout. In the bucket diagrams in this section, the amount/min of inulin at sites BS, P3, and U were always equal. In a similar fashion the amount/min of inulin at sites EFF, PC, and RV were always equal. If we add the amount/min of inulin found at the corresponding sites (BS + EFF; P3 + PC; U + RV), the sum must always equal the amount/min that entered the afferent arteriole

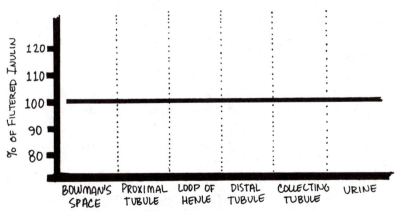

Figure 3. Inulin is neither secreted nor reabsorbed by the renal tubules. The amount of inulin filtered into Bowman's space is equal to the amount in the urine.

63

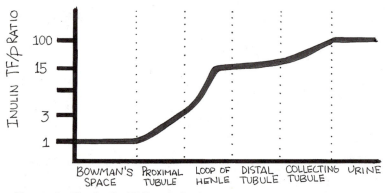

Figure 4. The inulin TF/P ratio in the renal tubules increases because water is reabsorbed.

at site AFF. This illustrates that no inulin is reabsorbed or secreted and that the amount/min filtered into the glomerulus is always equal to the amount/min excreted.

The concentration of inulin changes as it moves along the length of the renal tubule because water is reabsorbed (Figure 4). In the bucket diagrams this can be seen by the increase that occurs in the TF/P ratio for inulin along the length of the renal tubule. For example, at site BS the TF/P ratio is always be one for inulin (or any other freely filtered compound). At the end of the proximal tubule, the TF/P ratio is increased by the reabsorption of water that occurred in the proximal tubule. In the normal human kidney, approximately two-thirds of the filtered volume is reabsorbed by the end of the proximal tubule (site P3). This causes a three-fold increase in the concentration of inulin, although the amount/min of inulin has not changed as it moves through the proximal tubule. The TF/P ratio at site U is dependent upon the rate at which water is reabsorbed in the distal nephron. Water reabsorption is influenced by a number of factors—the state of hydration, for example—and can vary substantially. Because of this, the TF/P ratio at site U can also vary substantially from below 50 with high urine flow rates to over several hundred at low urine flow rates.

The TF/P ratio for inulin is of particular interest when we are attempting to determine if other compounds are being secreted or reabsorbed. If reabsorption of an unknown compound is occurring, the TF/P ratio for this compound will be lower than that of inulin. If

Inulin

	Plasma Concentration mg/ml	Filtered Load mg/min	Secreted mg/min	Reabsorbed mg/min	Excreted mg/min	Clearance
0.01						

	Plasma Concentration mg/ml						
	0.01	0.1	0.5	1.0	2.0	4.0	10.0
Filtered Load mg/min	1	10	50	100	200	400	1000
Secreted mg/min	–	–	–	–	–	–	–
Reabsorbed mg/min	–	–	–	–	–	–	–
Excreted mg/min	1	10	50	100	200	400	1000
Clearance	100	100	100	100	100	100	100

GFR = 100 ml/min

Table 1. As the plasma concentration of inulin increases, the filtered load and the amount of inulin excreted also increases. Inulin is neither secreted nor reabsorbed and this is not influenced by the plasma concentration. If GFR remains constant, the clearance of inulin also remains constant, despite the change in plasma concentration.

secretion of the unknown compound is occurring, the opposite will be true.

Increasing the plasma concentration of inulin does not effect the calculations we have discussed; however, this does not mean we can ignore the concentration of inulin. In fact, the plasma concentration must be known and maintained at a constant level for our calculations to be correct; however, the level we choose can vary without affecting the results. For example, if we double the plasma concentration of inulin (P_{in}) (Table 1), amount/min of inulin excreted ($U_{in} \times \dot{V}$) will double, and the calculation of GFR (clearance of inulin) will remain constant.

In most of the chapters in this book, we will see the influence of G-T balance on water reabsorption from the proximal tubule. Although G-T balance is not considered part of the renal concentrating mechanisms in general, alterations in proximal fluid and solute reabsorption can greatly influence body-fluid homeostasis. In a well-

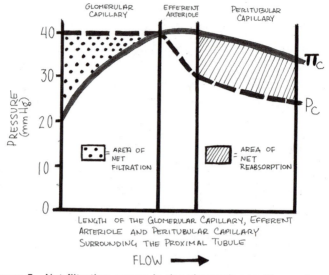

Figure 5. Net filtration occurs in the glomerular capillary, whereas net reabsorption occurs in the peritubular capillary.

hydrated individual, about two-thirds of the filtered volume is expected to be reabsorbed by the end of the proximal tubule. If the state of hydration remains normal, this percent of proximal reabsorption remains relatively constant despite changes in GFR. Several hypotheses are used to explain this observation. One of the most widely accepted hypotheses explains G-T balance as a balance in Starling forces that influence proximal water reabsorption. This hypothesis assumes that an increase in GFR results in an increase in protein concentration in the peritubular capillary surrounding the proximal tubule (see Figure 5). This elevated protein concentration increases oncotic pressure in the capillary, which in turn increases the Starling forces that favor fluid reabsorption from the proximal tubule, thus maintaining G-T balance at approximately two-thirds. This balance will be perturbed by alterations in the level of hydration. In a dehydrated person, G-T balance can increase significantly. This is thought to occur because peritubular capillary protein concentration (and thus oncotic pressure) is increased. This increased reabsorption of water from the proximal tubule helps to restore fluid homeostasis; however, it can also produce significant alterations in the transport of ions across the proximal tubule.

PAH EXCRETION

Introduction

Most of the para-aminohippuric acid (PAH) found in humans is highly bound to protein in the plasma; however, in our examples we consider only the unbound PAH. This PAH has several characteristics that make it useful to the clinician and renal physiologist. First, the unbound portion of PAH is freely filtered into Bowman's space across the glomerular capillary membrane. Second, PAH is rapidly transported by the P2 section of the proximal tubule. In fact, if the plasma concentration of PAH is low, this transport system is so effective that all of the unbound compound that enters the afferent arteriole is either filtered into Bowman's space or transported into the renal tubule. This means that the amount of unbound PAH in the peritubular capillary beyond the proximal tubule is zero. This secretion process most likely represents the kidney's effort to reduce the plasma concentration of a compound that is recognized as a potential toxin. Because bound PAH is not filtered in the glomerulus, secreted in the proximal tubule, or measured by normal means, we refer only to the unbound portion in this section.

Remember, we are ignoring splay in the bucket diagrams. The concept of splay is explained in the Corrections Section. If we increase the plasma concentration of PAH, we eventually exceed the ability of the transport system to secrete all of the unbound PAH from the capillary into the renal tubule. The maximum amount/min of PAH that can be transported has been calculated as 80 mg/min. For example, if 100 mg/min pass through the efferent arterioles, 80 mg/min are secreted into the proximal tubule and 20 mg/min remain in the peritubular capillaries and exit the kidney via the renal vein. Under these circumstances, the clearance of PAH does not equal renal plasma flow. Renal plasma flow can be calculated using PAH if we can determine the concentration of unbound PAH in the renal vein so that the Fick equation can be used (a slight error that exists in this calculation is discussed in the Corrections Section). The Fick equation can be used only when a compound is freely filtered and some of the compound is excreted.

Objectives

- Compare the filtration of PAH in the glomerulus to that of inulin.

- Explain why the clearance of PAH is equal to renal plasma flow (or effective renal plasma flow), if the PAH plasma concentration is low.

- Explain why the clearance of PAH decreases as the PAH plasma concentration increases above the transport maximum value.

- Graph the TF/P ratio for PAH in each section of the renal tubule.

- Explain how to calculate the TF/P ratio for PAH and explain why it differs from the TF/P ratio for inulin at most sites along the renal tubule.

- Explain transport maximum and show how it affects PAH clearance.

- Describe how PAH clearance might be used to estimate GFR.

- Hypothesize why your body secretes PAH.

- Identify the section of the renal tubule that secretes PAH and explain how this may occur.

- Calculate the various values listed in the examples and explain how they were calculated.

Example 1: Problem

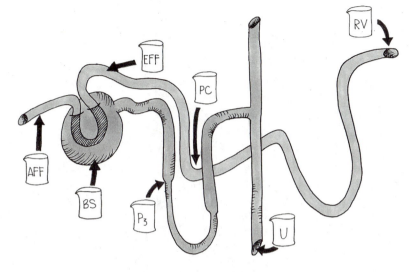

Site	Amount/min (mg / min)	Flow Rate (ml / min)	Concentration (mg / ml)	TF/P ratio
AFF		**500**	**0.1**	
BS		**100**		
EFF				
P3				
PC				
RV				
U		**1**		

G-T balance _____ **2/3** _____

Clearance _____

RPF _____

Extraction ratio _____

Filtration fraction _____

Tm _____ **80 mg/min**

Example 1: Solution

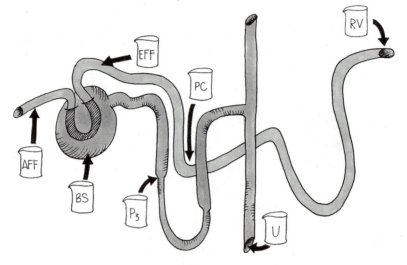

Site	Amount/min (mg / min)	Flow Rate (ml / min)	Concentration (mg / ml)	TF/P ratio
AFF	50	**500**	**0.1**	
BS	10	**100**	0.1	1
EFF	40	400	0.1	
P₃	50	33	1.5	15
PC	0	467		
RV	0	499	0	
U	50	1	50	500

G-T balance	2/3
Clearance	500
RPF	500
Extraction ratio	1
Filtration fraction	0.2
Tm	**80 mg/min**

Example 1: Explanation

The concentration at sites AFF, BS, and EFF is equal because unbound PAH is freely filtered. If you multiply the flow rate at sites AFF and BS by the concentration, you can determine the amount/min of PAH appearing at these two sites. If mass balance is to be maintained, the amount/min at site EFF is determined by subtracting the amount/min at site BS from the amount/min at site AFF. Similar calculations are made to determine the flow rate at site EFF.

The G-T balance is given as two-thirds. This means that two-thirds of the filtered volume (site AFF) is reabsorbed from the proximal tubule and that one-third remains in the proximal tubule and reaches site P3. Based upon these calculations, you can determine that of the 100 ml/min appearing at site BS (GFR), 33 ml/min reach the end of the proximal tubule and 67 ml/min are reabsorbed. The reabsorbed fluid is added to the flow rate found at site EFF so that the flow rate at site PC increases to 467 ml/min.

As with all freely filtered compounds, the TF/P ratio at site BS is one.

The transport maximum for PAH is given as 80 mg/min. The amount/min of PAH passing site EFF and entering the peritubular capillary adjacent to the proximal tubule is less than the transport maximum. This means that all of the PAH appearing at site EFF is secreted and added to the amount/min that entered the renal tubule by filtration into Bowman's space. This means that the amount/min of PAH appearing at site PC is zero and the amount/min of PAH at site P3 equals all of the PAH that entered the nephron at site AFF.

The TF/P ratio for PAH at site P3 is determined by dividing the concentration at site P3 by the concentration at site AFF.

No secretion of PAH occurs beyond the proximal tubule; therefore, all 50 mg/min that appeared at site P3 remain in the tubule and are found in the urine (site U). The concentration of PAH at site RV is zero because none of the compound is found in the renal vein. The concentration of PAH at site U is determined by dividing the amount/min of PAH at site U by the urine flow rate.

The TF/P ratio at site U is the concentration at site U divided by the concentration at site AFF.

The clearance of PAH is equal to RPF if we are below Tm and all PAH entering the nephron is excreted. Obviously, this is the case in this example. The clearance of PAH is equal to the amount/min of PAH excreted (site U) divided by the concentration of PAH in the afferent plasma (site AFF).

The extraction ratio for PAH is equal to the amount/min of PAH excreted, divided by the amount/min of PAH entering the nephron. In this example all the PAH is excreted; therefore, the extraction ratio is one. This can be calculated by dividing the difference between the concentration at site AFF and at site RV by the concentration at site AFF.

In this example, the flow rate at site BS is equal to GFR and the flow rate at site AFF is considered to equal RPF.

The filtration fraction is equal to GFR/RPF.

Example 2: Problem

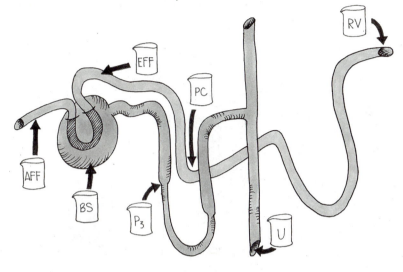

Site	Amount/min (mg / min)	Flow Rate (ml / min)	Concentration (mg / ml)	TF/P ratio
AFF		**400**	**0.1**	
BS		**100**		
EFF				
P3				
PC				
RV				
U		**1**		

G-T balance _____³/₄_____

Clearance _____

RPF _____

Extraction ratio _____

Filtration fraction _____

Tm _____**80 mg/min**_____

Example 2: Solution

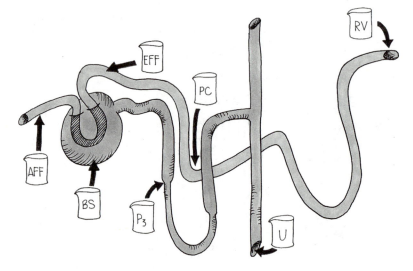

Site	Amount/min (mg / min)	Flow Rate (ml / min)	Concentration (mg / ml)	TF/P ratio
AFF	40	**400**	**0.1**	
BS	10	**100**	0.1	1
EFF	30	300	0.1	
P3	40	25	1.6	16
PC	0	375		
RV	0	399	0	
U	40	**1**	40	400

G-T balance	3/4
Clearance	400
RPF	400
Extraction ratio	1
Filtration fraction	0.25
Tm	**80 mg/min**

Example 2: Explanation

This example requires you to calculate the amount/min of PAH at sites AFF and BS. This is possible because you are given the flow rate at sites AFF and BS, and you know that unbound PAH is freely filtered and the concentration is the same at sites AFF, BS, and EFF. The flow rate at site EFF is determined by subtracting the flow rate at site BS from the flow rate at site AFF. The amount/min at site EFF is determined by subtracting the amount/min at site BS from the amount/min at site AFF or by multiplying the flow rate at site EFF by the concentration at site EFF.

The TF/P ratio at BS is always one for freely filtered compound such as PAH.

The G-T balance is given as three-fourths, which means that three-fourths of the filtered volume is reabsorbed in the proximal tubule. Based upon this, you can calculate that 75 ml/min are reabsorbed from the proximal tubule and that 25 ml/min reach site P3 at the end of the proximal tubule. The 75 ml/min that were reabsorbed are added to the 300 ml/min at site EFF so that 375 ml/min reach site PC.

The amount/min of PAH passing through site EFF is less than the transport maximum; therefore, all of the 30 mg/min at site EFF are secreted. The amount/min of PAH reaching the end of the proximal tubule (site P3) is 40 mg/min and no PAH is found at site PC. The concentration at site P3 is the amount/min found at this site divided by the flow rate. The TF/P ratio at site P3 is the concentration at this site divided by the concentration at site AFF.

The flow rate at site RV is calculated by subtracting the urine flow rate (site U) from the flow rate that entered the nephron (site AFF). This is possible because mass balance must be maintained.

The transport maximum for PAH is given as 80 mg/min. The amount/min of PAH passing through the peritubular capillaries adjacent to the proximal tubule is less than this transport maximum. Because of this, all of the PAH that entered the nephron is either filtered into Bowman's space or secreted into the proximal tubule and appears in the urine (site U).

The concentration of PAH at site U is calculated by dividing the amount/min at site U by the flow rate at site U.

The TF/P ratio for PAH at site U is equal to the urine concentration at site U divided by the concentration at site AFF.

The clearance of PAH is the amount/min of PAH excreted (site U) divided by the PAH concentration in the plasma (site AFF). The RPF is given (as the flow rate at site AFF); however, it should be noted that the clearance of PAH is equal to RPF because we are below the Tm for PAH and all PAH entering the nephron is excreted in the urine.

Extraction ratio is defined as the amount/min of a compound excreted divided by the amount/min entering the nephron. Obviously, in this example those amount/mins are equal; therefore, the extraction ratio will be one. Mathematically, this is determined by dividing the difference between the concentration at site AFF and site RV by the concentration at site AFF.

The filtration fraction is equal to GFR/RPF or 0.25.

Example 3: Problem

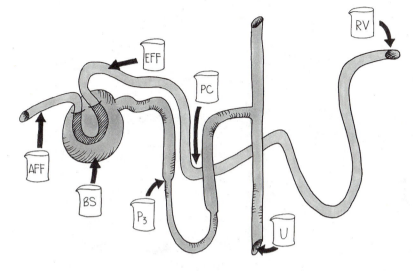

Site	Amount/min (mg / min)	Flow Rate (ml / min)	Concentration (mg / ml)	TF/P ratio
AFF			0.15	
BS		100		1
EFF				
P3				
PC		467		
RV				
U		2		

G-T balance _____ 2/3 _____

Clearance _____

RPF _____

Extraction ratio _____

Filtration fraction _____

Tm _____ **80 mg/min** _____

Example 3: Solution

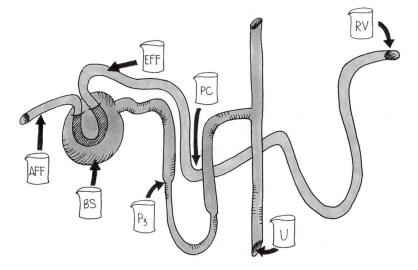

Site	Amount/min (mg / min)	Flow Rate (ml / min)	Concentration (mg / ml)	TF/P ratio
AFF	75	500	**0.15**	
BS	15	**100**	0.15	1
EFF	60	400	0.15	
P3	75	33	2.3	15
PC	0	**467**		
RV	0	498	0	
U	75	**2**	37.5	250

G-T balance   **2/3**

Clearance   500

RPF   500

Extraction ratio   1

Filtration fraction   0.20

Tm   **80 mg/min**

Example 3: Explanation

The plasma concentration of PAH at site AFF is given. Unbound PAH is freely filtered; therefore, the concentration of PAH must be the same at sites AFF, BS, and EFF.

The G-T balance is given as two-thirds. This means that two-thirds of the volume filtered into Bowman's space (site BS) is reabsorbed from the proximal tubule and that one-third appears at the end of the proximal tubule (site P3). Based upon this information, you can calculate that 33 ml/min appear at site P3. You are given that 467 ml/min appear at site PC in the peritubular capillary adjacent to site P3. If mass balance is to be maintained, 500 ml/min must have entered the nephron at site AFF. If 500 ml/min appear at site AFF, then the flow rate at site EFF is 400 ml/min because you are told that 100 ml/min appeared at site BS.

With this knowledge you can determine that 75 mg/min of PAH appear at site AFF, 15 mg/min at site BS, and 60 mg/min at site EFF. These values are determined by multiplying the flow rate at each site by the concentration (0.15 mg/ml).

The TF/P ratio for PAH (or any freely filtered compound) at site BS is one.

The transport maximum for PAH is given as 80 mg/min. The amount/min of PAH passing through the peritubular capillaries adjacent to the proximal tubule is less than this value; therefore, all of the PAH in the peritubular capillaries is secreted into the proximal tubule. The amount/min of PAH at site P3 equals the amount/min of PAH at site AFF. This is because all of the PAH entering the nephron is either filtered into Bowman's space or secreted into the renal tubule. All of the PAH appears at site P3; therefore, the amount/min appearing at site PC is zero.

The concentration of PAH at site P3 is calculated by dividing the amount/min of PAH at site P3 by the flow rate appearing at site P3. The TF/P ratio for PAH at site P3 is calculated by dividing the concentration at site P3 by the concentration at site AFF.

The flow rate of the urine is given as 2 ml/min. This means that the flow rate appearing at site RV must be the difference between this flow rate and the flow rate entering the nephron at site AFF (500 ml/min – 2 ml/min = 498 ml/min).

The amount/min of PAH at site RV is zero; therefore, the amount/ min at site U must be 75 mg/min. If the urine flow rate is 2 ml/min, the concentration of PAH in the urine must be 37.5 mg/ml.

The TF/P ratio at site U is 250. This is calculated by dividing the concentration of PAH at site U by the concentration of PAH at site AFF.

Clearance of PAH is the amount/min of PAH excreted (site U) divided by the PAH concentration in the plasma (site AFF).

RPF was calculated earlier based on the assumption of mass balance; however, you can also determine RPF by calculating the clearance of PAH. This is possible because PAH is below its transport maximum and all the unbound PAH entering the nephron is excreted in the urine.

If all the PAH entering the nephron is excreted, the extraction ratio is one. This is calculated by dividing the difference between the concentration of PAH and the afferent arteriole (site AFF) and the concentration in the renal vein (site RV) by the concentration in the afferent arteriole (site AFF).

Filtration fraction is equal to GFR/RPF.

Example 4: Problem

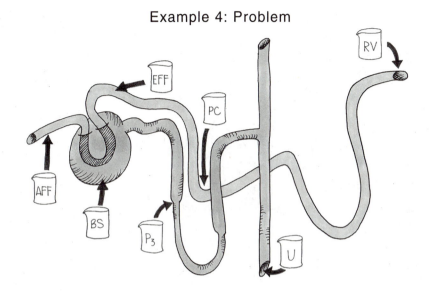

Site	Amount/min (mg / min)	Flow Rate (ml / min)	Concentration (mg / ml)	TF/P ratio
AFF		**500**	**0.3**	
BS				
EFF				
P3		**33**		
PC				
RV		**499**		
U				

G-T balance _____ **2/3** _____

Clearance _____

RPF _____

Extraction ratio _____

Filtration fraction _____

Tm _____ **80 mg/min** _____

Example 4: Solution

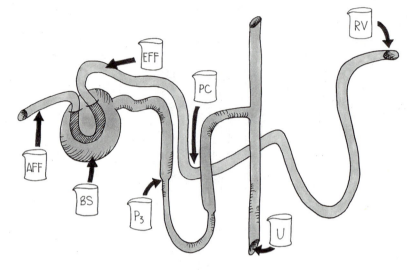

Site	Amount/min (mg / min)	Flow Rate (ml / min)	Concentration (mg / ml)	TF/P ratio
AFF	150	**500**	**0.3**	
BS	30	100	0.3	1
EFF	120	400	0.3	
P3	110	**33**	3.3	11
PC	40	467		
RV	40	**499**	0.08	
U	110	1	110	367

G-T balance _____ ²/₃ _____

Clearance _____ 367 _____

RPF _____ 500 _____

Extraction ratio _____ 0.73 _____

Filtration fraction _____ 0.20 _____

Tm _____ **80 mg/min** _____

82

Example 4: Explanation

Like all freely filtered compounds, the concentration of unbound PAH is the same at sites AFF, BS, and EFF. This also means that the TF/P ratio for PAH at site BS is one. You are given that RPF (the flow rate at site AFF) is 500 ml/min. If you multiply the flow rate at site AFF by the concentration at site AFF, you can calculate the amount appearing at site AFF per minute.

You are given that the G-T balance is two-thirds. This means that two-thirds of the filtered volume is reabsorbed from the proximal tubule and that one-third reaches the end of the proximal tubule (site P3). You are given that the flow rate at site P3 is 33 ml/min. With this information you can calculate that the flow rate at site BS (GFR) is 100 ml/min.

The amount/min of PAH at site BS is now calculated by multiplying the concentration at site BS by the flow rate at site BS. The flow rate and amount/min at site EFF is calculated by subtracting the appropriate values at site BS from those at site AFF.

You are given that the maximum amount/min of PAH that can be secreted by the proximal tubule (transport maximum) is 80 mg/min. In this example you can see that the amount/min of PAH passing through the peritubular capillaries adjacent to the proximal tubule (between site EFF and site PC) is greater than 80 mg/min. Because of this, not all the PAH is secreted into the renal tubule and some PAH remains at site PC. This is calculated by subtracting transport maximum from the amount/min appearing at site EFF (120 mg/min − 80 mg/min = 40 mg/min).

This means that the amount/min appearing at site P3 is the amount/min appearing at site BS plus the 80 milligrams that are secreted into the proximal tubule. No transport of PAH occurs beyond the end of the proximal tubule; therefore, the amount/min appearing at site P3 also appears at site U and the amount/min appearing at site PC appears at site RV.

The concentration at site RV equals the amount/min appearing at site RV (40 mg/min) divided by the flow rate at site RV (given as 499 ml/min). The flow rate at site U is equal to the difference between the flow rate that entered the nephron (site AFF) and the flow rate of site RV. The TF/P ratio at site U is equal to the concentration at site U divided by the concentration at site AFF.

The G-T balance is given in this example.

The clearance of PAH is equal to the amount of PAH excreted per minute divided by the concentration of PAH in the afferent arteriole (site AFF). Note that the clearance of PAH is not equal to renal plasma flow in this example because the transport maximum for PAH has been exceeded.

Renal plasma flow was given as the flow rate at site AFF. It can also be calculated using the Fick equation. To accomplish this, divide the amount/min of PAH excreted (site U) by the difference between the concentration and the afferent arteriole (site AFF) and the concentration in the renal vein (site RV).

Extraction ratio is equal to the amount/min excreted divided by the amount/min entering the nephron through the afferent arteriole. Mathematically, this is calculated by dividing the difference between the concentration and the afferent arteriole (site AFF) and the renal vein (site RV) by the concentration in the afferent arteriole (site AFF).

The filtration fraction is equal to GFR/ RPF.

The Tm for PAH is given as 80 mg/min.

Example 5: Problem

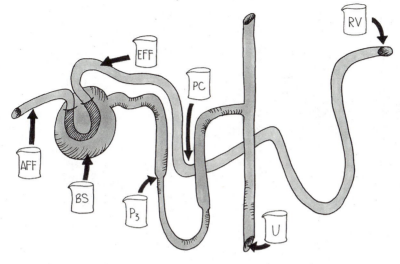

Site	Amount/min (mg / min)	Flow Rate (ml / min)	Concentration (mg / ml)	TF/P ratio
AFF				
BS	100	100		
EFF				
P3				
PC				
RV				
U		1		

G-T balance _____ **2/3** _____

Clearance _____

RPF _____

Extraction ratio _____

Filtration fraction ____ **0.20** _____

Tm _____ **80 mg/min** _____

Example 5: Solution

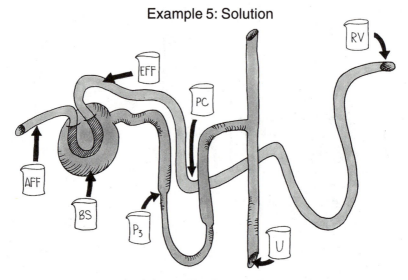

Site	Amount/min (mg / min)	Flow Rate (ml / min)	Concentration (mg / ml)	TF/P ratio
AFF	500	500	1	
BS	**100**	**100**	1	1
EFF	400	400	1	
P3	180	33	5.5	5.5
PC	320	467		
RV	320	499	0.64	
U	180	**1**	180	180

G-T balance _____ $2/3$ _____

Clearance _____ 180 _____

RPF _____ 500 _____

Extraction ratio _____ 0.36 _____

Filtration fraction _____ **0.20** _____

Tm _____ **80 mg/min** _____

Example 5: Explanation

The amount/min of PAH and the flow rate is given at site BS. With this information you can calculate the concentration at site BS (amount/min ÷ flow rate = concentration). You know that the concentrations at sites AFF, BS, and EFF are equal.

You are given that filtration fraction is 0.2. This means that GFR (flow rate at site BS) is 20% of RPF. With this information you can determine that RPF is 500 ml/min.

If the concentration at site AFF is 1 mg/min, the amount/min at site AFF is equal to 500 mg/min. If mass balance is to be maintained, the flow rate at site EFF must equal the flow rate at site AFF minus the flow rate at site BS. Using similar logic, the amount/min appearing at site EFF is also calculated by subtracting the appropriate values.

The amount/min of PAH appearing at site P3 equals the amount/min filtered at site BS plus the amount/min secreted into the proximal tubule. The amount/min filtered is 100 mg/min. The Tm for PAH has been exceeded; therefore, 80 mg/min are secreted. Added together this means 180 mg/min will be found at site P3.

The G-T balance is given as two-thirds. This means that two-thirds of a filtered volume is reabsorbed from the proximal tubule and one-third of this volume (or 33 ml/min) appears at the end of the proximal tubule (site P3). To maintain mass balance, we can assume that the flow rate at site PC is the difference between the flow rate entering the nephron and the flow rate appearing at site P3 (500 ml/min − 33 ml/min = 467 ml/min). You can also assume that the amount/min of PAH appearing at site PC is the difference between the amount/min entering the nephron and the amount/min appearing at site P_3 (500 mg/min − 180 mg/min = 320 mg/min).

The concentration at site P3 equals the amount/min at site P3 divided by the flow rate at site P3. The TF/P ratio at site P3 equals the concentration at site P3 divided by the concentration at site AFF.

The flow rate at site U is given as 1 ml/min. The flow rate at site RV is the difference between the flow rate entering the nephron and the flow rate appearing at site U.

No PAH is secreted beyond the end of the proximal tubule; therefore, the amount/min at site U equals the amount/min at site P3 and the amount/min at site RV equals the amount/min at site PC.

The concentration at site U is equal to the amount/min at site U divided by the flow rate at site U. The TF/P ratio at site U is the concentration at site U divided by the concentration at site AFF.

G-T balance is given as two-thirds.

The clearance of PAH is the volume of plasma that originally contained the amount of PAH excreted per minute. In this example, the PAH clearance is 180 ml/min (the amount/min at site U divided by the plasma concentration at site AFF). The clearance of PAH is equal to RPF if we are below Tm for PAH; however, in this example we are above Tm. The calculation of RPF must be made using the Fick equation. This is equal to the amount/min of PAH (site U) divided by the difference between the concentration of PAH at site AFF and site RV.

The extraction ratio is the difference between the concentration at site AFF and site RV divided by the concentration at site AFF. This ratio is the amount/min of PAH excreted divided by the amount/min entering the nephron.

The filtration fraction is equal to GFR/RPF.

The Tm for PAH is given as 80 mg/min.

PAH EXCRETION

Example 6: Problem

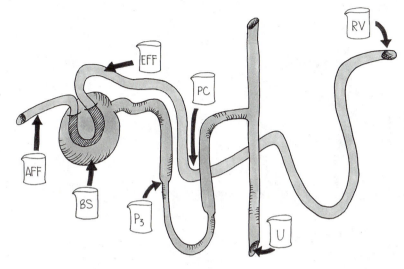

Site	Amount/min (mg / min)	Flow Rate (ml / min)	Concentration (mg / ml)	TF/P ratio
AFF				
BS		100		
EFF	1200	400		
P3				
PC				
RV				
U		1		

G-T balance _____ **2/3** _____

Clearance _____

RPF _____

Extraction ratio _____

Filtration fraction _____

Tm _____ **80 mg/min** _____

Example 6: Solution

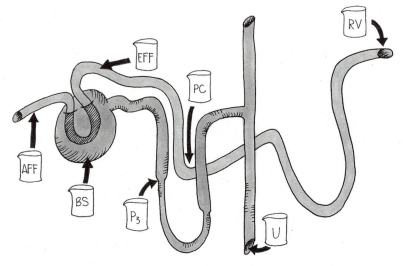

Site	Amount/min (mg / min)	Flow Rate (ml / min)	Concentration (mg / ml)	TF/P ratio
AFF	1500	500	3	
BS	300	**100**	3	1
EFF	**1200**	**400**	3	
P3	380	33	11.5	3.8
PC	1120	467		
RV	1120	499	2.24	
U	380	**1**	380	127

G-T balance ___**2/3**___

Clearance ___127___

RPF ___500___

Extraction ratio ___0.25___

Filtration fraction ___0.20___

Tm ___**80 mg/min**___

Example 6: Explanation

The amount/min of PAH at site EFF is given as 1200 mg/min and the flow rate at site EFF is 400 ml/min. By dividing, you can determine that the concentration is 3 mg/ml. You must remember that the concentration of any freely filtered compound is the same at sites AFF, BS, and EFF. For this same reason, the TF/P ratio at site BS is one as it is for any freely filtered compound.

The flow rate at site BS is given as 100 ml/min. To maintain mass balance, the flow rate at site AFF must equal the flow rate at site BS plus the flow rate at site EFF or, in this example, 500 ml/min. With this information you can multiply the flow rate at sites AFF and BS by the concentration to determine the amount/min of PAH appearing at each site .

The G-T balance is given as two-thirds, which means that two-thirds of the filtered volume is reabsorbed from the proximal tubule and that one-third reaches the end of the proximal tubule (site P3). You are given that GFR (the flow rate at site BS) is 100 ml/min; therefore, the flow rate at site P3 must be 33 ml/min. The flow rate at site PC is equal to the flow rate at site AFF minus the flow rate at site P3.

Tm for PAH has been exceeded. This means that the amount/min of PAH reaching site P3 is the amount/min filtered into Bowman's space (300 mg/min) plus the maximum amount/min of PAH that can be transported by the proximal tubule (80 mg/min). With this information, you can calculate the concentration of PAH at site P3 (380 mg/min ÷ 33 ml/min = 11.5 mg/ml). The TF/P ratio at site P3 is equal to the concentration appearing at site P3 divided by the concentration appearing in the afferent arteriole (site AFF). In this example, the TF/P ratio is 3.8 (11.5 mg/ml ÷ 3 mg/ml).

If mass balance is to be maintained, the amount/min of PAH at site PC must equal the amount/min tentering the nephron minus the amount/min appearing at site U.

PAH is only secreted in the proximal tubule; therefore, the amount/min at site U must equal the amount/min at site P3 and the amount/min at site RV must equal the amount/min at site PC.

The flow rate at site U is given as 1 ml/min. The flow rate at site RV must equal the flow rate entering the nephron minus the flow rate at site U (500 ml/min – 1 ml/min = 499 ml/min). With this information you can now calculate the concentration at site RV by dividing the amount/min at site RV by the flow rate at site RV. Similar calculations are used to provide the concentration at site U.

The TF/P ratio at site U is the concentration at site U divided by the concentration in the afferent arteriole.

G-T balance is given as two-thirds.

The clearance of PAH is calculated by dividing the amount/min of PAH excreted in the urine by the plasma concentration of PAH in the afferent arteriole (site AFF). The clearance value of PAH is no longer equal to RPF because we have exceeded Tm for PAH.

RPF is calculated using the Fick equation which is equal to the amount/min of PAH excreted divided by the difference between PAH concentration in the afferent arteriole (site AFF) and the concentration in the renal vein (site RV).

The extraction ratio for PAH is equal to the difference between the concentration and the afferent arterioles (site AFF) and the renal vein (site RV) divided by the concentration at site AFF.

The filtration fraction is equal to GFR/RPF.

Summary

It is well known that renal plasma flow can be estimated using the clearance of PAH. This is true only if the concentration of PAH in the plasma is low and its transport maximum has not exceeded. If these criteria are met, all of the PAH that enters the nephron will be excreted in the urine and the concentration in the renal vein should be zero.

Unfortunately, what you were told in the last paragraph is not totally true. Even at low plasma concentration, some unbound PAH will appear in the renal vein because some of the plasma that enters the kidney does not pass by a functional nephron. The PAH contained in this plasma cannot be extracted. This volume of plasma accounts for 10-15% of all the plasma flow that enters the kidney. As a result, the clearance of PAH is said to equal effective renal plasma flow (ERPF). ERPF is usually 10-15% less than RPF. To calculate true RPF, we must be able to measure the concentration of PAH in the renal vein. If we can accomplish this, we can then use the Fick equation, which measures all the plasma flow or RPF. This error in calculation is discussed in the Corrections Section. It should also be remembered that we have neglected to consider splay. This concept is also considered in the Corrections Section.

The plasma concentration of inulin does not alter its clearance; however, this is not true for PAH. The reason for this difference resides in the way these two compounds are handled in the nephron. Inulin is able to enter the renal tubule only by way of filtration into Bowman's space from the glomerular capillary; thus, there is no transport maximum for inulin. As plasma concentration is increased, there is a proportional increase in the filtered amount/min. With PAH there is a similar increase in the amount/min filtered as plasma levels increase, but the secreted amount/min cannot exceed a set maximum value. This maximum value or transport maximum is not affected by plasma concentration. When the plasma concentration is high enough so that the amount/min of PAH being delivered to the peritubular capillaries adjacent to the proximal tubule exceeds its transport maximum, the clearance value for PAH starts to drop. If we continue to increase the PAH concentration in the plasma, clearance of PAH will approach the clearance of inulin. This can be seen in Figure 6.

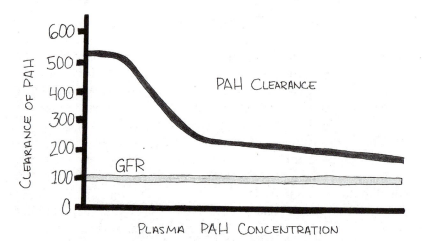

Figure 6. PAH clearance decreases when the amount of PAH in the peritubular capillary surrounding the proximal tubule exceeds the transport maximum. This occurs as the plasma concentration increases.

The values provided in Table 2 also illustrate this same point. The filtered load increases proportionally to plasma concentration; however, the amount/min being secreted will not exceed 80 mg/min. If you compare the values in Table 2 to Table 1 in the section for inulin, you will find that the amount/min filtered (filtered load) is the same for similar plasma concentrations in both examples. However, at the lower plasma concentrations, most of the excreted PAH enters the renal tubule by the process of secretion. It is this secretion that makes the PAH concentration greater than the inulin clearance. In both the inulin example and PAH example, 100 ml/min of plasma were cleared by filtration; however, in the PAH example an additional 400 ml/min of plasma were cleared by the process of secretion.

PAH

Plasma Conc. mg/ml	0.05	0.1	0.15	0.5	1.0	5.0	25
Filtered Load mg/min	5	10	15	50	100	500	2500
Secreted mg/min	20	40	60	80	80	80	80
Reabsorbed	–	–	–	–	–	–	–
Excreted mg/min	25	50	75	130	180	580	2580
Clearance	500	500	500	260	180	116	103

(GFR = 100 ml/min)

Table 2. As the plasma concentration of PAH increases, the filtered load and the amount of PAH excreted also increases. The amount of PAH secreted increases until transport maximum is reached and then remains constant. The clearance of PAH decreases after Tm is exceeded. The values in the table ignore splay. A discussion of splay is found in the Corrections Section.

At higher plasma concentrations, most of the excreted PAH enters the renal tubule by the process of filtration. In fact, at the uppermost concentration shown in Table 2, 100 ml/min were cleared by filtration and only 3 ml/min were cleared by secretion. The values at the right-hand side of this table compare to the right-hand side of Figure 6.

GLUCOSE EXCRETION

Introduction

Glucose is the product that is derived from the break down of much of the food we consume. Our body uses glucose for the production of energy in most tissues. Obviously, it would be counterproductive for our kidneys continually to excrete the glucose the rest of our body needs. To excrete low molecular weight compounds by filtration and yet retain glucose, our body has developed a cotransport system that reabsorbs the glucose that is initially filtered into Bowman's space. Like all noncharged, low molecular weight compounds, glucose appears in the glomerular filtrate at a concentration equal to that found in the afferent arteriole. Under normal conditions, the reabsorption process for glucose in the proximal tubule is so efficient that effectively no glucose is excreted in the urine. Glucose is reabsorbed with sodium in a cotransport mechanism that uses the Na^+-K^+ - ATPase energy developed on the basolateral membrane of the renal tubular cell. The details of this cotransport system are beyond the scope of this workbook; however, you should be able to find a description in most renal physiology texts.

The reabsorption of glucose continues throughout the length of the proximal tubule. The maximum amount/min of glucose that can be reabsorbed by both human kidneys is 375 mg/min. Once this transport maximum is reached, any additional glucose that is filtered in the glomerulus appears in the urine. Because of splay, some glucose appears in the urine before the filtered load of glucose reaches the Tm. The initial appearance of glucose in the urine occurs when the plasma glucose concentration reaches its renal threshold or approximately 180 mg/dl. The concept of splay is not considered in the problems in this section but is explained in the Corrections Section.

Several other interesting phenomena occur when we consider glucose excretion. For example, if the kidney did not metabolize any glucose, the concentration of glucose in the renal vein would exceed the concentration of glucose in the afferent arteriole under normal conditions. This occurs because all of the glucose appearing in the afferent arteriole also appears in the renal vein; however, because some of the plasma was used to form urine, the concentration of glucose increases in the renal vein. The higher concentration of glucose in the renal vein will cause the calculated extraction ratio to become negative. Another anomaly occurs if glucose is used to calculate renal plasma flow using the Fick equation. This is discussed in the Corrections Section.

Objectives

- Explain why glucose clearance is zero at low plasma concentration and why it increases as plasma glucose concentration increases.

- Compare the filtration of glucose in the glomerulus to that of PAH and inulin.

- Explain why the Fick equation cannot be used with glucose to calculate RPF in normal situations.

- Explain how the transport maximum affects glucose clearance.

- Hypothesize why your body reabsorbs glucose and explain what happens if this reabsorption does not occur.

- Construct a graph to show TF/P ratio in various segments of the renal tubule. Explain how this graph changes if the plasma concentration of glucose is increased.

- Determine the various values requested in the examples and explain how they were calculated.

- Explain why glucose can act as an osmotic diuretic if it is not reabsorbed in the proximal tubule.

Example 1: Problem

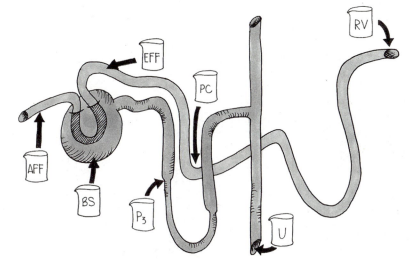

Site	Amount/min (mg / min)	Flow Rate (ml / min)	Concentration (mg / ml)	TF/P ratio
AFF	500	500		
BS		100		
EFF				
P3				
PC				
RV				
U		1		

G-T balance _____ **2/3** _____

Clearance _____

RPF _____

Extraction ratio _____

Filtration fraction _____

Tm _____ **375 mg/min** _____

GLUCOSE EXCRETION

Example 1: Solution

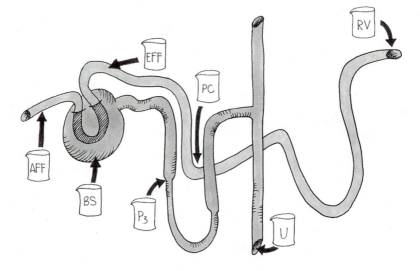

Site	Amount/min (mg / min)	Flow Rate (ml / min)	Concentration (mg / ml)	TF/P ratio
AFF	**500**	**500**	1	
BS	100	**100**	1	1
EFF	400	400	1	
P3	0	33	0	0
PC	500	467		
RV	500	499	1	
U	0	**1**	0	0

G-T balance _____ $^2/_3$ _____

Clearance _____ 0 _____

RPF _____ 500 _____

Extraction ratio _____ 0 _____

Filtration fraction _____ 0.20 _____

Tm _____ **375 mg/min** _____

Example 1: Explanation

The concentration of glucose at site AFF is determined by dividing the amount/min of glucose at site AFF by the flow rate of fluid at site AFF. Glucose is a freely filtered compound; therefore, the concentration at sites AFF, BS, and EFF is equal. The amount/min of glucose at site BS is determined by multiplying the concentration at site BS by the flow rate at site BS. The flow rate at site EFF and the amount/min at site EFF is determined by subtracting the appropriate value at site BS from the corresponding value at site AFF. Glucose is a freely filtered compound, therefore the TF/P ratio at site BS is equal to one.

The G-T balance is given as two-thirds, which means that two-thirds of the filtered flow rate is reabsorbed from the proximal tubule and one-third (or 33 ml/min) reaches the end of the proximal tubule (site P3). The 67 ml/min that are reabsorbed from the proximal tubule are added to the 400 ml/min that appeared at site EFF resulting in a flow rate of 467 ml/min at site PC.

You are given that glucose has a Tm of 375 mg/min, which means that up to 375 mg/min can be reabsorbed from the proximal tubule. The amount/min of glucose appearing at site BS (filtered load) is less than the transport maximum; therefore, the entire filtered load (100 mg/min) is reabsorbed. No glucose appears at site P3 and all of the glucose that entered the nephron (500 mg/min) appears at site PC.

The urine flow rate is given as 1 ml/min. This means that the remainder of the flow rate that entered the nephron (site AFF) appears at site RV. Because there is no reabsorption of glucose between site PC and RV, the amount/min of glucose appearing at site RV is the same at site PC.

Because no glucose appeared at either site P3 or site U, the concentration at each site is zero and the TF/P ratio is also zero at both sites.

The clearance of glucose is equal to the volume of plasma that originally contained the amount of glucose excreted per minute. Because no glucose is excreted, the clearance of glucose must be equal to zero.

The flow rate appearing at site AFF (RPF) is given as 500 ml/min.

The extraction ratio for glucose is zero. (In fact, the extraction ratio is slightly negative because the concentration of glucose is higher in the renal vein than in the renal artery. This is discussed in the Corrections Section).

The filtration fraction is equal to GFR (flow rate at site BS) divided by RPF (flow rate at site AFF). Both values are given.

The transport maximum is given as 375 mg/min.

Example 2: Problem

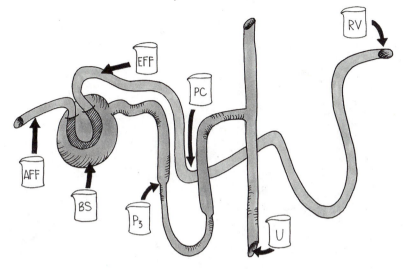

Site	Amount/min (mg / min)	Flow Rate (ml / min)	Concentration (mg / ml)	TF/P ratio
AFF	**1500**	**500**		
BS				
EFF				
P3		**33**		
PC				
RV				
U		**1**		

G-T balance _____

Clearance _____

RPF _____

Extraction ratio _____

Filtration fraction __**0.20**_____

Tm _____**375 mg/min**____

Example 2: Solution

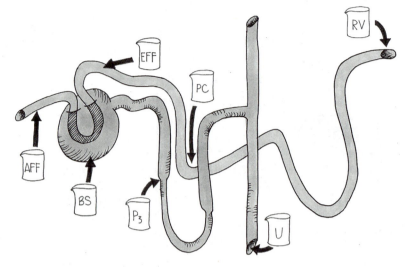

Site	Amount/min (mg / min)	Flow Rate (ml / min)	Concentration (mg / ml)	TF/P ratio
AFF	1500	500	3	
BS	300	100	3	1
EFF	1200	400	3	
P3	0	33	0	0
PC	1500	467		
RV	1500	499	3	
U	0	1	0	0

G-T balance __2/3__

Clearance __0__

RPF __500__

Extraction ratio __0__

Filtration fraction __0.20__

Tm __375 mg/min__

Example 2: Explanation

The concentration of glucose at site AFF is equal to the amount/min at site AFF divided by the flow rate at site AFF. Glucose is freely filtered into Bowman's space and appears at sites AFF, BS, and EFF at the same concentration. The TF/P ratio for glucose at site BS is equal to one, as with any freely filtered compound.

The filtration fraction is given as 0.2. This means that 20% of RPF (flow rate at site AFF) appears as glomerular filtrate (site BS). From this information, you can determine that GFR (flow rate at site BS) is 100 ml/min. The amount/min at site BS is determined by multiplying the concentration and the flow rate at this site.

The amount/min at site EFF is the difference between the amount/min at site AFF and the amount/min at site BS. The flow rate at site EFF is calculated using the same logic.

You are given that 33 ml/min appear at the end of the proximal tubule (site P3). This means that 67 ml/min of the flow rate that was filtered at site BS (GFR) is reabsorbed in the proximal tubule. To maintain mass balance, the flow rate at site PC must equal the flow rate at site EFF plus the reabsorbed volume (400 ml/min + 67 ml/min = 467 ml/min).

The filtered load (amount/min at site BS) is less than the Tm for glucose; therefore, all of the filtered glucose is reabsorbed from the proximal tubule. The amount/min of glucose at site P3 is therefore zero and all the glucose that entered the nephron appears at site PC. This total reabsorption of glucose from the proximal tubule causes the concentration of glucose at site P3 to be zero and the TF/P ratio of glucose is also zero.

You are given that the urine flow rate is 1 ml/min; therefore, the flow rate appearing at site RV must be 499 ml/min or the difference between the excreted flow rate and the flow rate entering the nephron per minute.

All of the glucose entering the nephron appears at site RV. The concentration of glucose at site RV is equal to the amount/min appearing at site RV divided by the flow rate at site RV. The concentration of glucose at site U is zero and the TF/P ratio at site U is also zero.

G-T balance is equal to the ratio of fluid reabsorbed from the proximal tubule (between sites BS and P3) and the filtered flow rate (site BS). You can calculate that the reabsorbed flow rate is 67 ml/min or two-thirds of GFR (site BS).

The clearance of glucose is zero because no glucose remains in the urine and all appears in the plasma at site RV.

You are given that RPF (site AFF flow rate) is 500 ml/min.

The extraction ratio is zero because no glucose is excreted.

You are given that the filtration fraction is 0.20 and that the Tm for glucose is 375 mg/min.

GLUCOSE EXCRETION

Example 3: Problem

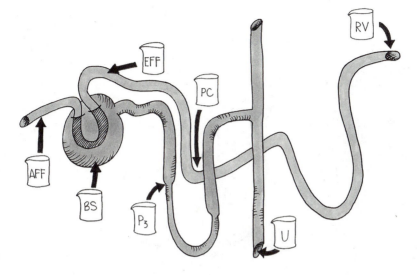

Site	Amount/min (mg / min)	Flow Rate (ml / min)	Concentration (mg / ml)	TF/P ratio
AFF	**2000**		**4**	
BS		**100**		
EFF				
P3				
PC				
RV				
U		**1**		

G-T balance _____ **2/3** _____

Clearance _____

RPF _____

Extraction ratio _____

Filtration fraction _____

Tm _____ **375 mg/min** _____

Example 3: Solution

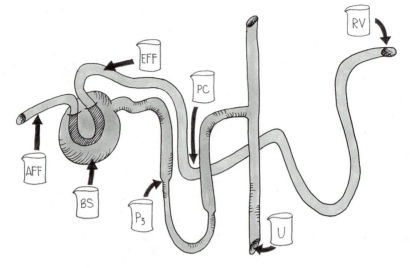

Site	Amount/min (mg / min)	Flow Rate (ml / min)	Concentration (mg / ml)	TF/P ratio
AFF	**2000**	500	**4**	
BS	400	**100**	4	1
EFF	1600	400	4	
P3	25	33	0.76	0.19
PC	1975	467		
RV	1975	499	3.96	
U	25	**1**	25	6.25

G-T balance _____ $^2/_3$ _____

Clearance _____ 6.25 _____

RPF _____ 500 _____

Extraction ratio _____ 0.01 _____

Filtration fraction _____ 0.20 _____

Tm _____ **375 mg/min** _____

Example 3: Explanation

The concentration of glucose appearing at sites AFF, BS, and EFF is equal because glucose is freely filtered in the glomerulus. The flow rate at site AFF is calculated by dividing the amount/min at site AFF (2000 mg/min) by the concentration (4 mg/ml). The amount/min at site BS is determined by multiplying the concentration at site BS and the flow rate at this site.

The TF/P ratio at site BS is equal to one as it is for all freely filtered compounds.

The flow rate and amount/min appearing at site EFF are determined by subtracting the appropriate values at site BS from those at site AFF. This is possible because mass balance must be maintained between these sites.

You are given that G-T balance is two-thirds, which means that one-third of the filtered flow rate appearing at site BS (GFR) appears at the end of the proximal tubule (site P3) and two-thirds is reabsorbed. The reabsorbed flow rate is added to that found at site EFF so that 467 ml/min appears at site PC.

You are given that the Tm for glucose is 375 ml/min and you calculated that the filtered load is 400 mg/min. This means that 25 mg/min of the filtered load appears at site P3 and 375 mg/min is reabsorbed. This amount/min that is reabsorbed is added to the amount/ min found in the efferent arteriole (site EFF) and increases the amount/min appearing at site PC to 1975 mg/min. The concentration of glucose at site P3 (0.76 mg/ml) is the amount/min at site P3 (25 mg/min) divided by the flow rate at site P3 (33 ml/min). The TF/P ratio at site P3 is the concentration at this site divided by the concentration at site AFF.

We assume that no glucose is reabsorbed beyond the end of the proximal tubule; therefore, all of the glucose appearing at site P3 is excreted (site U). The concentration at site U is determined by dividing the amount/ min at site U (25 mg/min) by the flow rate at site U (1 ml/min). The TF/P ratio at site U is the concentration at site U divided by the concentration at site AFF.

The concentration of glucose at site RV is slightly less than the concentration of glucose at site AFF because glucose is present in the urine.

The G-T balance value is given.

The clearance of glucose is equal to the amount/min excreted divided by the plasma concentration at site AFF.

RPF is equal to the plasma flow rate calculated for site AFF.

In theory, the Fick equation could be used to calculate RPF in this example because some glucose is being excreted in the urine. For this to be accurate, the kidney could not use or manufacture any glucose; however both occur, which makes this a questionable assumption.

The extraction ratio is equal to the difference between the concentration at site AFF and site RV divided by the concentration at site AFF and has a positive value.

The filtration fraction is equal to GFR/RPF. In this example it is 0.20.

The Tm for glucose is given as 375 mg/min.

GLUCOSE EXCRETION

Example 4: Problem

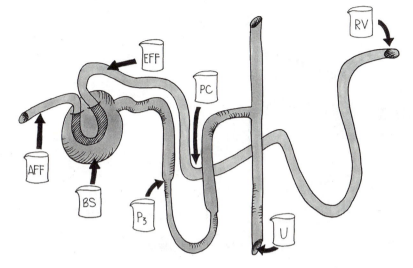

Site	Amount/min (mg / min)	Flow Rate (ml / min)	Concentration (mg / ml)	TF/P ratio
AFF	**2500**	**500**		
BS				
EFF				
P3	125			
PC				
RV				
U		1		

G-T balance   2/3

Clearance _____

RPF _____

Extraction ratio _____

Filtration fraction   **0.20**

Tm _____

Example 4: Solution

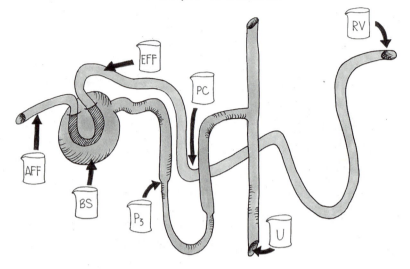

Site	Amount/min (mg / min)	Flow Rate (ml / min)	Concentration (mg / ml)	TF/P ratio
AFF	**2500**	**500**	5	
BS	500	100	5	1
EFF	2000	400	5	
P3	125	33	3.79	0.76
PC	2375	467		
RV	2375	499	4.76	
U	125	1	125	25

G-T balance _____ $^2/_3$ _____

Clearance _____ 25 _____

RPF _____ 500 _____

Extraction ratio _____ 0.048 _____

Filtration fraction _____ **0.20** _____

Tm _____ 375 mg/min _____

Example 4: Explanation

The concentration of glucose at site AFF can be determined by dividing the amount/min at site AFF by the flow rate at site AFF. Glucose is freely filtered; therefore, the concentration at sites AFF, BS, and EFF are equal and the TF/P ratio at site BS is one.

The filtration fraction is 0.20. This means that 20% of the plasma entering the nephron (site AFF) appears as GFR (flow rate at site BS or 100 ml/min). The amount/min at site BS equals the concentration at site BS multiplied by the flow rate at site BS.

The amount/min at site EFF and the flow rate at site EFF can be determined by subtracting the appropriate values at site BS from the corresponding values at site AFF.

The G-T balance is given as two-thirds. This means that two-thirds of GFR (flow rate at site BS) is reabsorbed from the proximal tubule and that one-third (33 ml/min) appears at site P3. The concentration of glucose at site P3 is determined by dividing the amount/min of glucose appearing at site P3 by the flow rate appearing at site P3. The TF/P ratio at site P3 is equal to the concentration at site P3 divided by the concentration at site AFF.

The amount/min of glucose appearing at site PC equals the amount/min of glucose that appeared in the efferent arteriole (site EFF) plus the amount/min reabsorbed from the proximal tubule. The flow rate of plasma appearing at site PC equals the flow rate at site EFF plus the volume reabsorbed from the proximal tubule. You are given that two-thirds of the filtered volume is reabsorbed from the proximal tubule; therefore, the flow rate appearing at site EFF is 467 ml/min.

The urine flow rate is given as 1 ml/min. This means that the flow rate of plasma appearing at site RV must be the difference between the flow rate entering the nephron (site AFF) and the urine flow rate.

We assume that glucose is not transported beyond the end of the proximal tubule; therefore, the amount/min of glucose appearing at site U equals the amount/min at site P3, and the amount/min at site RV equals the amount/min at site PC. The concentration of glucose at site RV is equal to the amount/min of glucose appearing at site RV divided by the flow rate appearing at site RV. The concentration of glucose at site U is equal to the amount/min appearing at site U divided by the urine flow rate. The TF/P ratio for glucose is equal to the concentration of glucose at site U divided by the concentration at site AFF.

You are given that the G-T balance is two-thirds.

The clearance of glucose in this example is a positive value and is equal to the amount of glucose excreted per minute divided by the concentration at site AFF.

You are given that RPF (the flow rate appearing at site AFF) is 500 ml/min.

The extraction ratio also is positive. The extraction ratio is equal to the difference between the concentration of glucose at site AFF and the concentration of glucose at site RV divided by the concentration of glucose at site AFF.

Filtration fraction is given as 0.20.

In this example, you are asked to calculate Tm for glucose. The Tm for glucose is equal to the amount/min that can be reabsorbed by the proximal tubule. This is the difference between the filtered load (amount/min appearing at site BS) and the amount/min reaching the end of the proximal tubule (amount/min appearing at site P3).

Example 5: Problem

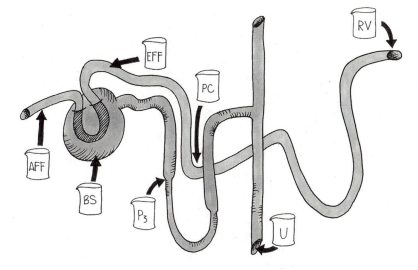

Site	Amount/min (mg / min)	Flow Rate (ml / min)	Concentration (mg / ml)	TF/P ratio
AFF	**2800**	**400**		
BS		**100**		
EFF				
P3	**350**			
PC				
RV				
U		**2**		

G-T balance _____ **3/4** _____

Clearance _____

RPF _____

Extraction ratio _____

Filtration fraction _____

Tm _____

Example 5: Solution

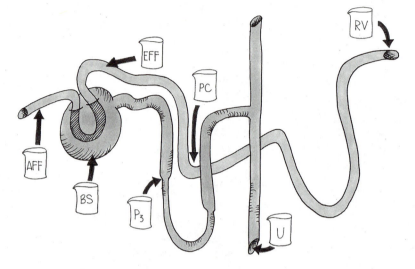

Site	Amount/min (mg / min)	Flow Rate (ml / min)	Concentration (mg / ml)	TF/P ratio
AFF	**2800**	**400**	7	
BS	700	**100**	7	1
EFF	2100	300	7	
P3	**350**	25	14	2
PC	2450	375		
RV	2450	398	6.16	
U	350	**2**	175	25

G-T balance _____ **3/4** _____

Clearance _____ 50 _____

RPF _____ 400 _____

Extraction ratio _____ 0.12 _____

Filtration fraction _____ 0.25 _____

Tm _____ 350 mg/min

Example 5: Explanation

You are given that the flow rate of plasma appearing at site AFF is 400 ml/min and the amount/min of glucose appearing at site AFF is 2800 mg/min. By dividing the amount/min by the flow rate, you can determine that the concentration at site AFF is 7 mg/ml. Glucose is a freely filtered compound; therefore, the concentration at sites AFF, BS, and EFF are equal. The TF/P ratio at site BS is equal to one as it is for all freely filtered compounds. You are given that GFR (flow rate at site BS) is 100 ml/min. If you multiply this flow rate by the concentration, you can determine that 700 mg/min appear at site BS. If you subtract the amount/min and flow rate values at site BS from the appropriate values at site AFF, you can determine the amount/min of glucose and the flow rate of plasma that appears at site EFF. This is possible because mass balance must be maintained between these three locations.

You are given that G-T balance is three-fourths, which means that three-fourths of the flow rate appearing at site BS (GFR) is reabsorbed from the proximal tubule and one-fourth appears at site P3. You are given that 350 mg/min of glucose appears at site P3 . By dividing this amount/min by the flow rate appearing at site P3, you can determine that the concentration of glucose at site P3 is 14 mg/ml. The TF/P ratio for glucose at site P3 equals the concentration of glucose at site P3 divided by the concentration of glucose at site AFF.

The amount/min of glucose appearing at site PC equals the difference between the amount/min entering the nephron at site AFF and the amount/min appearing in the tubule at site P3. The flow rate appearing at site PC equals the difference between the flow rate entering the nephron and the flow rate appearing at site P3.

You are given that the urine flow rate is 2 ml/min. To maintain mass balance, the flow rate appearing at site RV must equal the difference between the flow rate entering the nephron at site AFF and the flow rate excreted as urine.

We assume that no glucose is transported beyond the end of the proximal tubule. This means that the amount/min of glucose appearing at site RV equals the amount/min appearing at site PC, and the amount/min appearing at site U equals the amount/min appearing at site P3. The concentration at site RV is determined by dividing the amount/min appearing at site RV by the flow rate of plasma at site RV. The concentration at site U equals the amount/min appearing at site U divided by the urine flow rate (flow rate at site U). The TF/P ratio at site U equals the concentration at site U divided by the concentration at site AFF.

You are given that G-T balance is three-fourths.

The clearance of glucose equals the amount/min excreted in the urine (amount/min at site U) divided by the concentration of glucose in the fluid entering the nephron at site AFF.

You are given that renal plasma flow (the flow rate at site AFF) is 400 ml/min.

The extraction ratio equals the difference between the concentration at site AFF and the concentration at site RV divided by the concentration at site AFF.

The filtration fraction is equal to GFR/RPF.

The Tm for glucose is equal to the maximum amount/min that can be reabsorbed from the proximal tubule per minute. This is equal to the difference between the amount/min appearing at site BS (filtered load) and the amount/min excreted in the urine (amount/min at site U).

Summary

Glucose, like inulin and unbound PAH is freely filtered and appears in Bowman's space (site BS) at the same concentration as it appeared in the plasma at sites AFF and EFF. The reabsorption of glucose in the proximal tubule is rapid and much of the filtered load is reabsorbed by the end of the early segment (P1). In the P1 segment, glucose is reabsorbed in a 1 to 1 ratio with sodium. In the P3 segment of the proximal tubule, the ratio is 1 to 3. Although more energy is required to reabsorb a molecule of glucose, this reabsorption process allows the concentration of glucose in the tubular fluid to be lowered to near zero under normal conditions.

As mentioned previously, the bucket diagrams do not account for splay. In reality, splay significantly lowers the plasma concentration at which glucose appears in the urine. The concept of splay is discussed in the Corrections Section.

Figure 7 illustrates the change in the amount/min of glucose seen at different segments along the proximal tubule. Assuming that the filtered load is in a normal range, no glucose is found beyond the end of the proximal tubule. However, when the filtered load exceeds the ability of the proximal tubule to reabsorb all of the glucose, some

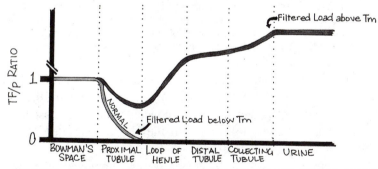

Figure 7. Normally, all the filtered glucose is reabsorbed in the proximal tubule; therefore, the TF/P ratio decreases to zero by the end of the P3 segment. If the amount of filtered glucose excedes Tm, some glucose will reach the end of the proximal tubule. The glucose TF/P ratio in the remainder of the renal tubule will increase as water is reabsorbed. The actual glucose TF/P value at any point along the tubule is less than the inulin TF/P ratio and depends upon several factors. These factors include the rate of water reabsorbtion, the amount of glucose that enters the descending loop of Henle, and any glucose that might be reabsorbed along the more distal segments of the nephron.

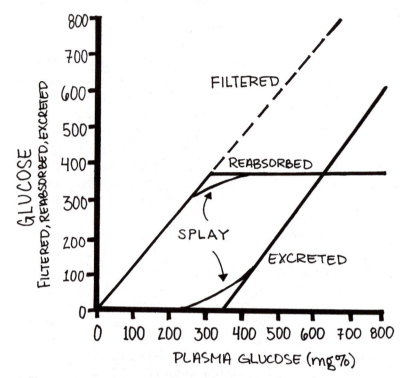

Figure 8. As plasma glucose concentration changes, the amount of glucose filtered, reabsorbed, and excreted per minute is illustrated. GFR is considered to remain constant at 100 ml/min. The influence of splay, which produces a gradual change in the amount of glucose reabsorbed and excreted is also illustrated. Splay is discussed in the Corrections Section.

glucose is found beyond site P3 and enters the descending limb of the loop of Henle. As the fluid moves through the remainder of the kidney, water reabsorption will cause the concentration of glucose to increase. This can be seen by comparing the TF/P ratio at site P3 to the TF/P at site U in glucose examples 4 or 5.

The clearance of glucose is normally zero; however, when glucose is excreted the clearance value becomes positive. As the plasma concentration of glucose is increased, the clearance of glucose approaches the appearance of inulin.

Table 3 also demonstrates this fact. As the plasma concentration is increased, the filtered load is increased at a proportional rate. Once the transport maximum for glucose is exceeded, any further increase in the filtered load results in an equal amount/min of glucose

Glucose

Plasma Conc. mg/ml	0.5	1.0	3.0	5.0	6.0	10.0	20.0
Filtered Load mg/min	50	100	300	500	600	1000	2000
Secreted mg/min	–	–	–	–	–	–	–
Reabsorbed mg/min	50	100	300	375	375	375	375
Excreted mg/min	0	0	0	125	225	625	1625
Clearance	0	0	0	25	37.5	62.5	81.25

(GFR = 100 ml/min)

Table 3. As the plasma concentration of glucose increases, the filtered load increases in the same manner as inulin or PAH. The amount filtered equals the amount reabsorbed until the transport maximum is reached. As the plasma glucose concentration continues to increase, the amount reabsorbed remains constant and the kidney begins to excrete glucose in increasing amounts. These examples disregard the effect of splay. Splay is discussed in the Corrections Section.

appearing in the urine. This excreted glucose carries water with it, which results in an increased urinary flow rate. The first symptom noted by patients with diabetes mellitus is often an increased fluid consumption as their body attempts to replace the increased fluid lost in the urine.

URINE CONCENTRATING MECHANISMS

Introduction

The mammalian kidney contains only M-type nephrons, which are capable of making a concentrated urine. The kidneys of birds have some "M"or mammalian-type nephrons and can therefore excrete a slightly hypertonic urine. Other vertebrates are forced to maintain body-fluid homeostasis using different mechanisms. These other mechanisms have included decreasing glomerular size (or totally eliminating the glomerulus), maintaining high circulating levels of solute, excreting uric acid to reduce urinary water loss, and regulating the excretion of salt through special glands that help maintain an appropriate body fluid concentration and volume. Although each of these mechanisms is quite effective in a given environment, the mammalian nephron accomplishes the task in a unique fashion that allows this group of animals to live in a wide variety of environments without the necessity of extrarenal glands or other mechanisms to maintain body-fluid homeostasis.

The urine diluting and concentrating capabilities of the mammalian nephron have long been recognized; however, the mechanisms through which these events are accomplished have been difficult to explain. The basic description of the countercurrent multiplication system was published in the 1940s and represented a major breakthrough in our understanding of the urinary concentrating process. A more precise explanation of the system was published in the 1970s, which helped explain the role of urea recycling in the development of the inner medullary gradient. The subcellular mechanisms involved in the reabsorption of solute from the thick ascending limb of the loop of Henle were described in the 1980s. These advancements have helped us develop a working knowledge of the urinary concentrating process. Briefly, the essential factors of this mechanism include: 1) movement of water out of the descending limb of the loop (and possibly some solute movement into the tubule), 2) impermeability of the ascending limb to water, 3) passive sodium movement out of the thin ascending limb and passive urea movement into the tubule, 4) sodium transport out of the thick ascending limb by both active transport on the basolateral membrane and secondary active

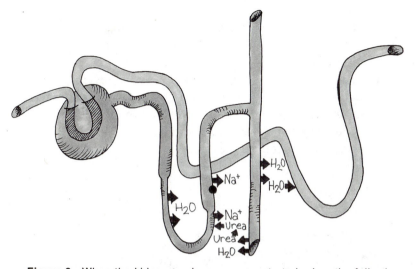

Figure 9. When the kidney produces a concentrated urine, the following events occur along the nephron: 1) water is reabsorbed from the descending loop of Henle because the surrounding interstitial fluid is hyperconcentrated; 2) sodium is reabsorbed passively down its concentration gradient in the thin ascending loop of Henle; 3) sodium is actively reabsorbed from the thick ascending loop of Henle; 4) under the influence of ADH, water is reabsorbed from the distal tubule, collecting tubule, and collecting duct; and 5) under the influence of ADH, urea is reabsorbed from the intramedullary collecting duct. Urea contributes approximately 50% of the intramedullary osmotic gradient. Some of the urea that is reabsorbed from the collecting duct passively enters the thin ascending loop of Henle.

transport on the lumenal membrane, 5) the regulation of water (and perhaps urea) permeability in the collecting duct by ADH, and 6) removal of water from the inner medullary region of the kidney by the vasa recta. Some of these mechanisms are well established experimentally, whereas others represent only our best understanding of the how the process must function. These basic characteristics are shown in Figure 9.

The examples in this chapter are based on our knowledge of the renal countercurrent multiplication system and its role in the development of a concentrated urine. Examples are given in which the plasma concentration of antidiuretic hormone (ADH) are low, normal, or high. As in the previous examples, the data are extrapolated from current knowledge and cannot be obtained (or validated) experimentally using current techniques. It is possible that experts in the area may dispute given values; however, the basic concepts provided in these examples would be agreed upon by most knowledgeable individuals.

The bucket diagrams for these examples have several new locations identified on these figures. The new sites were required to explain more fully the mechanisms involved in the countercurrent multiplication system. The new sites are TLH, DCT, CCT, PCD, and IS. The locations for all the sites are:

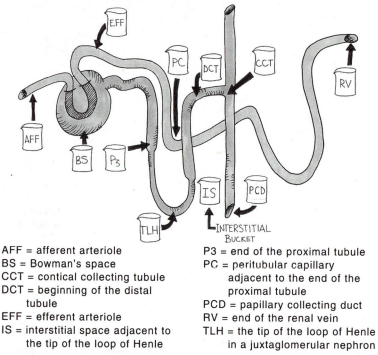

AFF = afferent arteriole
BS = Bowman's space
CCT = contical collecting tubule
DCT = beginning of the distal
    tubule
EFF = efferent arteriole
IS = interstitial space adjacent to
    the tip of the loop of Henle

P3 = end of the proximal tubule
PC = peritubular capillary
    adjacent to the end of the
    proximal tubule
PCD = papillary collecting duct
RV = end of the renal vein
TLH = the tip of the loop of Henle
    in a juxtaglomerular nephron

The information requested in each problem has also changed from what was requested in the previous examples. You are asked to calculate the fluid concentration (mOsm/kg H_2O) at each tubular site, the flow rate (ml/min), inulin concentration (mg/ml), inulin TF/P ratio, osmolal clearance, and free-water clearance. The inulin values allow us to determine the sites along the nephron where water reabsorption occurs because the inulin concentration in the renal tubule (and thus inulin TF/P ratio) changes only because of water transport.

The purpose of the renal concentrating mechanism is to maintain fluid homeostasis by excreting filtered water in the overhydrated person or returning filtered water to the renal vein in the dehydrated person. The measure of how well this is accomplished is called free-water clearance. Free-water clearance is defined as the volume of pure water that must be added to or subtracted from one minute of urine production to make the concentration of that urine equal to the plasma concentration. Free-water clearance is calculated by subtracting osmolal clearance from urine flow rate. Osmolal clearance is calculated as for any compound. Briefly, the urine concentration (expressed in mOsm/kg H_2O) is multiplied by the urine flow rate and this product is then divided by the plasma concentration (expressed in mOsm/kg H_2O). When free-water clearance is negative, hyperosmotic urine is excreted, and when free-water clearance is positive, hypotonic urine is excreted. If free-water clearance is zero, then the urine osmolal concentration is equal to the osmolal concentration of plasma.

In some examples you are asked to calculate the number of milliosmoles appearing in the urine or in the renal vein. This presents a problem because osmolality is expressed in units per kg H_2O, whereas flow is expressed in liters. To simplify this issue assume that 1 liter of plasma is equal to 1 kg of H_2O.

Objectives

- Explain why the loop of Henle is a countercurrent multiplication system.

- Describe the movement of solutes and water in the descending limb of the loop of Henle.

- Explain why water is reabsorbed from the descending limb of the loop of Henle.

- Explain why the inulin TF/P ratio is the same at the tip of the loop of Henle and at the end of the thick ascending limb.

- Explain the differences that occur in the renal vein osmolal concentration when ADH level is low, normal, and high.

- Be able to calculate the flow rate of fluid at any site along the renal tubule if you know GFR and the inulin TF/P ratio at that segment.

- Explain why the urine concentration is equal to the inner medullary concentration when ADH levels are elevated but less than the interstitial concentration when ADH levels are low.

- Explain osmolal clearance.

- Explain the concept of free-water clearance.

Example 1 – Normal ADH: Problem

Site	Fluid Concentration mOsm/kg H$_2$O	Flow Rate (ml / min)	Inulin Concentration (mg / ml)	Inulin TF/P ratio
AFF	300	500	1	
BS		100		
EFF	302			
P3				3
PC	300			
TLH	600		6.25	
DCT	150			
CCT	300		12	
PCD	600	1.5		
IS	600			
RV				

Osmolal clearance _____

Free-water clearance _____

127

Example 1 – Normal ADH: Solution

Site	Fluid Concentration mOsm/kg H$_2$O	Flow Rate (ml / min)	Inulin Concentration (mg / ml)	Inulin TF/P ratio
AFF	300	500	1	
BS	300	100	1	1
EFF	302	400	1	
P3	300	33	3	3
PC	300	467		
TLH	600	16	6.25	6.25
DCT	150	16	6.25	6.25
CCT	300	8.3	12	12
PCD	600	1.5	66.7	66.7
IS	600			
RV	299	498.5	0.80	

Osmolal clearance   3 ml/min

Free-water clearance   – 1.5 ml/min

Example 1– Normal ADH: Explanation

The fluid concentration, flow rate, and inulin concentration is given for site AFF. Inulin is freely filtered in the glomerulus; therefore, its concentration is the same at sites AFF, BS, and EFF. The flow rate is given for site BS. The fluid concentration at site BS is considered to equal the fluid concentration at site AFF because the compounds that determine plasma osmolality are primarily small and are freely filtered, appearing in the glomerular filtrate at the same concentration as the plasma (The mOsm/kg H_2O concentration at site BS may be slightly less than that of the fluid in the glomerular capillary because of the Gibbs-Donnan equilibrium. This difference is miniscule and is ignored in this example.) the mOsm/kg H_2O concentration of plasma increases as it moves through the glomerulus; therefore, the mOsm/kg H_2O concentration of the fluid in Bowman's space equals that of the incoming plasma, but is less than the mOsm/kg H_2O concentration of the plasma leaving the glomerular capillary.

The flow rate at site EFF is calculated by subtracting the flow rate at site BS from the flow rate at site AFF.

The mOsm/kg H_2O concentration of the fluid at site EFF is slightly greater than the mOsm/kg H_2O concentration at site AFF because the protein that remains in the plasma becomes more concentrated as water is filtered into Bowman's space. In this example, the concentration at site EFF is given as 302 mOsm/kg H_2O.

The inulin TF/P ratio is given as 3 at site P3. This means that the inulin concentration at site P3 is three times greater than it is in Bowman's space; therefore, the inulin concentration also will be 3. If the inulin concentration at site P3 increases three times, then two-thirds of the filtered water reabsorbed in the proximal tubule. Of the 100 ml filtered into Bowman's space at site BS, 33 ml/min appear at site P3 and 67 ml/min are reabsorbed into the peritubular capillary. The 67ml/min that are reabsorbed are added to the flow rate at site EFF (400 ml/min) so that 467 ml/min appears at site PC. Fluid reabsorption in the proximal tubule is isosmotic. Therefore, the concentration of fluid at site P3 and site BS are equal. This value is approximately equal to the fluid concentration at site PC; thus the fluid concentration at site P3 and site PC is 300 mOsm/kg H_2O.

You are given that the inulin concentration at site TLH is 6.25 mg/ml. The inulin TF/P ratio at site TLH equals the inulin concentration at site TLH divided by the inulin concentration at site AFF; for this example the ratio is 6.25. The flow rate at site TLH is calculated by dividing the TF/P ratio at site TLH into GFR (remember that GFR is equal to the flow rate at site BS) ($100 \div 6.25 = 16$). The fluid concentration at site TLH is given as 600 mOsm/kg H_2O. The ascending limb of the loop of Henle is impermeable to water; therefore, the flow rate, inulin concentration, and inulin TF/P ratio at site DCT must equal that at site TLH. Sodium is passively reabsorbed from the thin ascending limb and actively reabsorbed from the thick ascending limb of the loop of Henle. Because of this, the fluid mOsm/kg H_2O concentration at site DCT is hyposmotic under normal conditions. In this example, you are given that it equals 150 mOsm/kg H_2O.

The inulin concentration at site CCT is given as 12 mg/ml. This means that some water is reabsorbed between site DCT and site CCT. The TF/P ratio at site CCT equals the inulin concentration at site CCT divided by the inulin concentration at site AFF. The flow rate appearing at site CCT is calculated by dividing GFR by the TF/P ratio at site CCT. Based on this calculation, the flow rate at site CCT is 8.3 ml/min. The concentration of the tubular fluid at site CCT is given as 300 mOsm/kg H_2O.

You are given that the flow rate of tubular fluid at site PCD is 1.5 ml/min. The TF/P ratio for inulin at site PCD can be determined by dividing this flow rate into GFR ($100 \div 1.5 = 66.7$). The concentration of inulin in the glomerular filtrate is 1; therefore, the inulin concentration at site PCD must be 66.7 mg/ml. You are given that the fluid concentration at site PCD and site IS is 600 mOsm/kg H_2O.

The flow rate at site RV is equal to the flow rate at site AFF minus the urine flow rate, which is measured at the end of the papillary collecting duct (site PCD). The inulin concentration at site RV is equal to the amount/min of inulin appearing at site RV divided by the flow rate at site RV. No inulin is secreted or reabsorbed by the renal tubule; therefore, the amount/min at site RV must be the difference between the amount/min at site AFF and the amount/min that was filtered into Bowman's space (site BS). This means that 400 mg/min of inulin appeared at site RV and the inulin concentration is 0.8 mg/ml ($400 \div 498.5$).

The mOsm/kg H_2O concentration of the fluid at site RV is equal to the number of milliosmoles appearing at the site divided by the flow rate. The number of milliosmoles is determined as the difference between the number of milliosmoles entering the nephron at site AFF and the number of milliosmoles excreted in the urine. The number of entering milliosmoles is equal to the fluid concentration at site AFF times the flow rate (in liters) at site AFF (300 mOsm/kg $H_2O \times 0.5$ liters/min = 150 milliosmoles/min). The number of milliosmoles lost in the urine is 600 mOsm/kg H_2O times the urine flow rate measured at site PCD (0.0015 liters/min) (remember 1 kg H_2O is assumed to equal 1 liter). Based on these calculations, it can be seen that 150 mOsm/ min entered the kidney and 0.9 mOsm/min were excreted. If the difference between these values is divided by the flow rate (expressed in liters) in the renal vein (site RV), the concentration of the fluid at site RV is approximately 29 9 mOsm/kg H_2O ($149.1 \div 0.4985 = 299$).

The osmolal clearance is calculated by multiplying the urine mOsm/kg H_2O concentration times the urine flow rate divided by the plasma mOsm concentration (600 mOsm/kg $H_2O \times 1.5$ ml/min) $\div$ 300 mOsm/kg H_2O = 3 ml/min). Free-water clearance is equal to the urine flow rate minus the osmolal clearance (1.5 ml/min – 3 ml/min = –1.5 ml/min).

Example 2 – Low ADH: Problem

Site	Fluid Concentration mOsm/kg H$_2$O	Flow Rate (ml / min)	Inulin Concentration (mg / ml)	Inulin TF/P ratio
AFF	300	500	1	
BS			1	
EFF	302	400		
P3			3	
PC	300			
TLH	600		6.25	
DCT	150			
CCT	300		6.7	
PCD	50	4		
IS				
RV				

Osmolal clearance   _____

Free-water clearance   _____

Example 2 – Low ADH: Solution

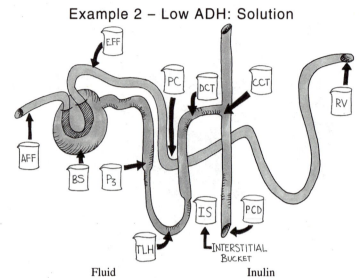

Site	Fluid Concentration mOsm/kg H$_2$O	Flow Rate (ml / min)	Inulin Concentration (mg / ml)	Inulin TF/P ratio
AFF	300	500	1	
BS	300	100	1	1
EFF	302	400	1	
P3	300	33	3	3
PC	300	467		
TLH	600	16	6.25	6.25
DCT	150	16	6.25	6.25
CCT	300	15	6.7	6.7
PCD	50	4	25	25
IS	600			
RV	302	496	0.8	

Osmolal clearance   0.67 ml/min

Free-water clearance   3.33 ml/min

Example 2 – Low ADH: Explanation

The inulin concentration at sites BS and AFF are given. Inulin is a freely filtered compound; therefore, the concentration at sites AFF, BS, and EFF must be equal. As with all freely filtered compounds the TF/P ratio for inulin at site BS is 1. The fluid mOsm/kg H_2O concentration and fluid flow rate at site AFF are given. Remember that the fluid mOsm/kg H_2O concentration at site BS is assumed to be equal to that at site AFF.

The fluid mOsm/kg H_2O concentration at site EFF increases slightly because water is filtered into Bowman's space thus concentrating proteins that remain behind in the plasma. The fluid flow rate at site EFF is given. The glomerular filtration rate (flow rate at site BS) is calculated by subtracting the flow rate at site EFF from the flow rate at site AFF.

You are given that the inulin concentration at site P3 is 3 mg/ml. This is three times greater than the plasma inulin concentration; therefore, you can calculate that the inulin TF/P ratio at site P3 is three. Because inulin is neither secreted nor reabsorbed by the renal tubule this increase occurs only because water is removed. To obtain a TF/P ratio of three, two-thirds of GFR is reabsorbed in the proximal tubule. This means that of the 100 ml filtered into Bowman's space (site BS), 33 ml reach the end of the proximal tubule (site P3). The 67 ml that are reabsorbed are added to the flow rate that appears at site EFF so that 467 ml appears at site PC. The fluid concentration at site P3 is given as 300 mOsm/kg H_2O, which is also approximately equal to the concentration at site PC.

The fluid concentration at site TLH is given as 600 mOsm/kg H_2O. You are also given that the inulin concentration is 6.25 mg/ml. Because the plasma concentration (site AFF) of inulin is 1 mg/ml, you can determine that the TF/P ratio at site TLH is 6.25. The flow rate appearing at site TLH is calculated by dividing the TF/P ratio for inulin at site TLH into GFR ($100 \div 6.25 = 16.0$).

You are given that the fluid concentration at site DCT is given as 150 mOsm/kg H_2O. No fluid is reabsorbed between site TLH and site DCT; therefore, the fluid flow rate, inulin concentration, and inulin TF/P ratio at site DCT must equal those for site TLH.

The fluid concentration at site CCT is given as 300 mOsm/kg H_2O. You are also given that the inulin concentration at site CCT is 6.7 mg/ml. This means that the TF/P ratio for inulin at site CCT is also 6.7. By dividing this TF/P ratio into GFR, you can determine that the flow rate at site CCT is 15 ml/min.

You are given that the fluid flow rate at site PCD is 4 ml/min. The TF/P ratio for inulin at any site is equal to the flow rate at that site divided into the GFR ($100 \div 4 = 25$). Because you know that the plasma concentration of inulin is one, the inulin concentration at site PCD must be 25 ml/min. You are given that the fluid concentration at site PCD is 50 mOsm/kg H_2O. The fluid concentration at site IS (adjacent to the tip of the loop of Henle) equals the fluid concentration at the tip of the loop of Henle or 600 mOsm/kg H_2O, because the membrane of the thin descending limb is highly permeable to water and therefore the fluid concentration in the tubule equilibrates with the fluid in the surrounding interstitial space.

The flow rate at site RV is the difference between the flow rate that entered the kidney (site AFF) and the urine flow rate (site PCD). The inulin concentration at site RV is determined by dividing the amount/min of inulin at site RV by the flow rate at site RV. Because you know the flow rate and concentration of inulin at site AFF, you can calculate that the amount/min of inulin present at site AFF is 500 mg/min. You know that the filtered load of inulin is 100 mg/min (100 ml/min × 1 mg/ml). Inulin is not transported by the renal tubule and the amount/min filtered is equal to the amount/min excreted. If 100 mg/min are excreted, then 400 mg/min must reach site RV. By dividing the amount/min of inulin reaching site RV by the flow rate of site RV, you can determine that the concentration of inulin at this site is approximately 0.8 mg/ml.

The mOsm/kg H_2O concentration of the tubular fluid appearing at site RV is the difference between the number of milliosmoles that entered the kidney and the number of milliosmoles that were excreted per minute. The number of milliosmoles entering the kidney equals 300 mOsm/kg H_2O × 0.5 L/min or 150 mOsm/min. The number of milliosmoles/min excreted equals 50 mOsm/kg H_2O × 0.004 L/min or 0.2 mOsm/min. This means that the fluid in the renal vein has a concentration of 302 mOsm/kg H_2O (149.8 mOsm/min ÷ 0.496 L/min = 302 mOsm/kg H_2O).

Osmolal clearance is equal to the urine mOsm/kg H_2O concentration times the urine flow rate divided by the plasma mOsm/kg H_2O concentration (50 mOsm/kg $H_2O \times$ 4 ml/min $\div$ 300 mOsm/kg H_2O = 0.67 ml/min). The free-water clearance is equal to the urine flow rate minus the milliosmole concentration (4 ml/min − 0.67 ml/min = 3.33 ml/min).

Example 3 – High ADH: Problem

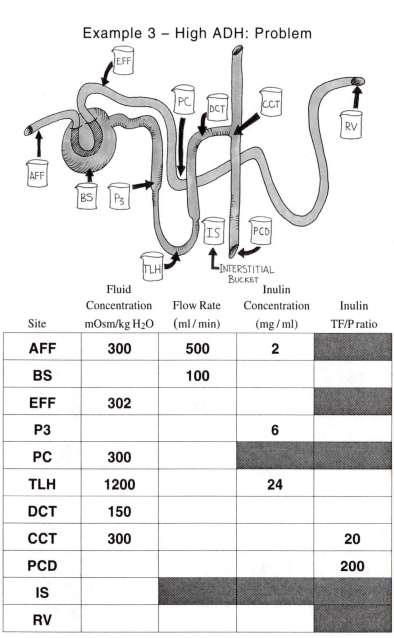

Site	Fluid Concentration mOsm/kg H₂O	Flow Rate (ml / min)	Inulin Concentration (mg / ml)	Inulin TF/P ratio
AFF	300	500	2	
BS		100		
EFF	302			
P3			6	
PC	300			
TLH	1200		24	
DCT	150			
CCT	300			20
PCD				200
IS				
RV				

Osmolal clearance _____

Free-water clearance _____

Example 3 – High ADH: Solution

Site	Fluid Concentration mOsm/kg H$_2$O	Flow Rate (ml / min)	Inulin Concentration (mg / ml)	Inulin TF/P ratio
AFF	**300**	**500**	2	
BS	300	**100**	2	1
EFF	**302**	400	2	
P3	300	33	**6**	3
PC	**300**	467		
TLH	**1200**	8.3	**24**	12
DCT	**150**	8.3	24	12
CCT	**300**	5	40	**20**
PCD	1200	0.5	400	**200**
IS	1200			
RV	299.1	499.5	1.6	

Osmolal clearance   2 ml/min

Free-water clearance   − 1.5 ml/min

Example 3 – High ADH: Explanation

You are given that the fluid concentration at site AFF is 300 mOsm/kg H_2O, the flow rate at site AFF is 500 ml/min, and the concentration of inulin at site AFF is 2 mg/ml. You know that inulin is freely filtered and has the same concentration at sites AFF, BS, and EFF. Because of this, inulin has a TF/P ratio at site BS of one. You are given GFR (the flow rate at site BS) is 100 ml/min. From these values, you can determine that the flow rate appearing at site EFF is 400 ml/min. The fluid mOsm/kg H_2O concentration at site BS is assumed to equal the fluid mOsm/kg H_2O concentration at site AFF (remember that the concentration at site BS is slightly less than that at site AFF because of the Gibbs-Donnan equilibrium effect). The fluid mOsm/kg H_2O concentration at site EFF is assumed to be elevated because the water that is filtered into the glomerulus concentrates the proteins that remain in the plasma.

The inulin concentration at site P3 is given as 6 mg/min. If you divide the inulin concentration at site TLH by the plasma inulin concentration (site AFF), you can determine that the TF/P ratio at site P3 is 3. The flow rate appearing at site P3 is determined by dividing the TF/P ratio for inulin at site P3 into the glomerular filtration rate (100 ml/min ÷ 3 = 33 ml/min). The fluid concentration at site P3 is equal to the fluid concentration at site BS or 300 mOsm/kg H_2O.

You are given that the fluid concentration at site PC is 300 mOsm/kg H_2O. The flow rate at site PC equals the flow rate at site EFF plus the flow rate reabsorbed from the proximal tubule (67 ml/min) or 467 ml/min.

The inulin concentration at site TLH is given as 24 mg/ml. If you divide this concentration by the plasma inulin concentration, the TF/P ratio for inulin at site TLH is 12. The flow rate appearing at site TLH is determined by dividing the TF/P ratio for inulin into GFR. Any change in inulin concentration must be due to water reabsorption because no inulin is transported by the renal tubules. You are given that the fluid concentration at site TLH is 1200 mOsm/kg H_2O.

The tubular membrane between site TLH and site DCT is impermeable to water; therefore, the flow rate, inulin concentration, and inulin TF/P ratio at site DCT must be equal to those values you calculated at site TLH. You are given that the fluid concentration at site DCT is 150 mOsm/kg H_2O.

The TF/P ratio for inulin is given as 20 at site CCT. The flow rate appearing at site CCT is determined by dividing this value into GFR (100 ml/min ÷ 20 = 5 ml/min). If the TF/P ratio is 20 at site CCT, the concentration of inulin at site CCT is determined by multiplying this TF/P ratio by the plasma concentration of inulin (20 × 2 ml/min = 40 ml/min). You are given that the fluid concentration at site CCT is 300 mOsm/kg H_2O.

This example refers to a condition of high ADH levels in the circulation; thus, water is rapidly reabsorbed from the collecting tubule, which results in a urine osmolality equal to that appearing at the tip of the loop of Henle or 1200 mOsm/kg H_2O. This mOsm/kg H_2O concentration must also be present at site IS.

High ADH levels make the membrane at site PCD highly permeable to H_2O; therefore the concentrations of fluid in site PCD (and the urine) will equal that of the interstitial space or 1200 mOsm/min. You are given that the TF/P ratio for inulin at site PCD is 200. The flow rate appearing at site PCD is calculated by dividing this TF/P ratio into GFR to determine that the urine flow rate is 0.5 ml/min. The inulin concentration in the urine (end of site PCD) is equal to the TF/P ratio at site PCD times the plasma concentration of inulin.

The flow rate appearing in the renal vein (site RV) is equal to the difference between urine flow rate and the flow rate that originally entered the nephron at site AFF. The inulin concentration at site RV equals the amount/min of inulin appearing at site RV divided by the flow rate appearing at site RV. The amount/min of inulin at site RV is equal to the difference between the amount/min that entered the nephron (site AFF) and the amount/min that was filtered into Bowman's space (site BS). The fluid mOsm/kg H_2O concentration at site RV is equal to the number of mOsm/min appearing at site RV divided by the flow rate appearing at site RV. The number of milliosmoles in the renal vein is equal to the difference between the number of milliosmoles that entered the nephron and the number of milliosmoles excreted in the urine per minute. The number of milliosmoles entering the nephron is calculated by multiplying the fluid mOsm/kg H_2O concentration at site AFF by the flow rate at site AFF (300 mOsm/kg H_2O × 0.5 L/min = 150 mOsm/min). The number of milliosmoles excreted per minute is equal to 1200 mOsm/kg H_2O times 0.0005 L/m or 0.6 mOsm/min. The difference between these two sites is 149.4 mOsm/kg H_2O. If this value is then divided by the flow rate appearing at site RV, you can determine the fluid mOsm/kg H_2O concentration at site RV (149.4 mOsm/kg H_2O mOsm/min ÷ 0.4995 L/min = 299.1 mOsm/kg H_2O).

The osmolal clearance is equal to the urine mOsm/kg H_2O concentration times the urine flow rate divided by the plasma mOsm/kg H_2O concentration (1200 mOsm/kg H_2O × 0.5 ml/min ÷ 300 mOsm/kg H_2O = 2 ml/min). The free-water clearance is equal to the urine flow rate minus the osmolal clearance (0.5 ml/min – 2 ml/min = –1.5 ml/min).

Summary

The examples provided in this section explain how the nephron helps to maintain body-fluid homeostasis. Despite the importance of the nephron in this process, many other factors are also involved. These include peripheral capillary permeability, physical and biochemical properties of cell membranes, hormonal regulation of solute and water movement, changes in fluid intake, insensible water loss, and loss of fluid and electrolytes through the gastrointestinal tract. These factors are beyond the scope of this chapter, but are important and must be addressed when evaluating fluid balance in patients.

Despite our greatly improved understanding of the renal concentrating system, several areas have not been fully explored. For example, our understanding of the countercurrent multiplication system has outstripped our knowledge of the countercurrent exchange that occurs in the vasa recta. Renal physiologists continue to disagree on the basic mechanisms used by the vasa recta to maintain solute hyperconcentration in the inner medullary region of the kidney. From what we now understand the purpose of this capillary network is to deliver nutrients to the inner medullary tissue and to remove the water that was reabsorbed from the descending loop of Henle and from the collecting duct from this region. Several hypotheses have been proposed to explain how this capillary system selectively removes more water than solute; however, none have been widely accepted. Understanding this mechanism represents a continuing challenge for both the renal physiologist and the student.

BODY FLUIDS

Introduction

A major task of our renal system is the regulation of body-fluid volume and concentration. In a healthy individual, this is achieved mainly by hormonal control over the reabsorption of sodium and water in the distal nephron. In disease conditions, following injury, or in extremely stressful environments, alterations in body-fluid balance can occur that overwhelm the kidney's ability to maintain homeostasis. Under these conditions, life threatening shifts in body-fluid volume and concentration can occur because of excessive loss or gain of solute, water, or both.

This chapter considers several conditions that produce shifts in body-fluid volume and concentration. So that you can understand clearly the consequences of any specific change in body fluid, only a single factor is changed at a time. In real-world situations, we are seldom this fortunate. Frequently, disease states alter solute and water balance simultaneously, thus compounding the complexity of patient diagnosis and treatment. Because of the importance of body-fluid homeostasis in the maintenance of health, our understanding of these issues is both challenging and important.

As in previous chapters, you will make assumptions that will make it easier to calculate the requested values. For example, you must assume that one kilogram of water is equal to one liter. In introductory chemistry, you learned that one liter of distilled water is equal to one kilogram at approximately $4^{\circ}C$. Obviously, body fluid is not distilled water and is not at $4^{\circ}C$. The presence of high molecular weight proteins and lipids in plasma replace water and alter the measured concentration of ionic compounds. Each liter of plasma contains only 930-940 ml of water; therefore, the concentration of sodium measured in plasma should be increased by 6-7% to give an accurate measure of this cation per liter of water.

The effect of temperature on the volume of a kilogram of water should be considered; however, the discrepancy produced by this alteration is minimal. At $37^{\circ}C$, the volume of one liter of water is expanded by approximately 0.6-0.7%; however, this small difference is not worthy of consideration.

In each example, two Darrow-Yannet diagrams (*Journal of Clinical Investigation* 14:266, 1935) are given. The ordinate (Y axis) represents the mOsm/kg H_2O concentration of the compartment and the abscissa (X axis) represents the volume contained in the intracellular (I) and extracellular (E) space. You are asked to draw Darrow-Yannet diagrams that illustrate the new body-fluid volume and concentration that should exist after the indicated alteration. You are also asked to supply the missing data in the table and are given enough information to make the necessary calculations.

The problems illustrate conditions that usually change the original condition in opposite directions. For example, you are asked to calculate the change in concentration and volume that exist after the loss of 1L of plasma and the gain of 1L of plasma. The effect each of these changes produces on the original condition should be considered separately except in Example 4. Example 4 first demonstrates the effect of dehydration and then considers the compounding effect of seawater ingestion in the dehydrated person.

Objectives

- Using a Darrow-Yannet diagram, graph the changes in concentration and volume that occur in the intracellular and extracellular compartments following: 1) plasma loss, 2) addition of isotonic saline to the plasma, 3) increased sodium concentration in the plasma, 4) decreased sodium concentration in the plasma, 5) hypotonic dehydration, 6) overhydration, and 7) dehydration plus ingestion of seawater.

- Calculate the total number of milliosmoles in intracellular and extracellular compartments if given the necessary information.

- Calculate the change in plasma mOsm/kg H_2O concentration following changes in fluid or solute concentration.

- Explain why the concentration of the intracellular compartment and the concentration of the extracellular compartment remain constant under a variety of conditions.

- Explain why drinking seawater will harm a dehydrated person.

- Calculate the intracellular volume to total body volume ratio and explain how this ratio can be changed by ingestion of salt, loss of salt, or ingestion of seawater.

Example 1: Problem

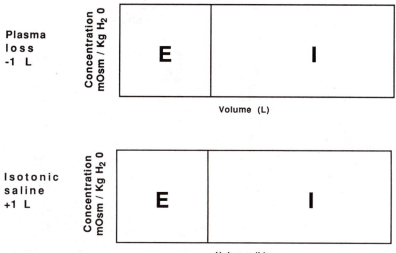

Plasma loss -1 L

Concentration mOsm / Kg H₂0

E   I

Volume (L)

Isotonic saline +1 L

Concentration mOsm / Kg H₂0

E   I

Volume (L)

	Original	Original − 1 L of Plasma	Original + 1L of Isotonic saline
Total volume (L)	45		
Extracellular volume (L)	15		
Intracellular volume (L)			
Extracellular vol / Total volume			
Intracellular vol / Total volume			
mOsm/kg H₂O	290		
Total mOsm			
Extracellular mOsm			
Intracellular mOsm			

Example 1: Solution

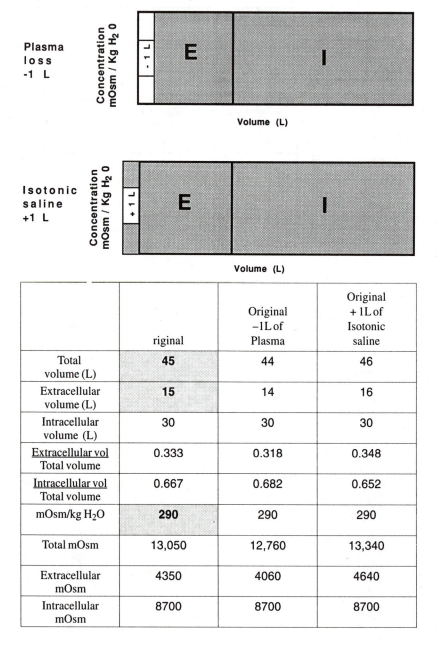

	riginal	Original −1L of Plasma	Original + 1L of Isotonic saline
Total volume (L)	45	44	46
Extracellular volume (L)	15	14	16
Intracellular volume (L)	30	30	30
Extracellular vol / Total volume	0.333	0.318	0.348
Intracellular vol / Total volume	0.667	0.682	0.652
mOsm/kg H₂O	290	290	290
Total mOsm	13,050	12,760	13,340
Extracellular mOsm	4350	4060	4640
Intracellular mOsm	8700	8700	8700

Example 1: Explanation

In Example 1, the total volume of the patient is given as 45 L and that extracellular volume is 15 L. By subtracting these two values, you can determine that intracellular volume is 30 L. If you divide the extracellular volume and the intracellular volume by the total volume, you can determine that the ratio for each is 0.333 and 0.667 respectively (obviously, the sum of these two ratios must equal one).

You are given the concentration of the body fluid as 290 mOsm/kg H_2O. By multiplying this concentration by the total body volume, you can determine that the total number of milliosmoles in the body is 13,050. If you multiply the extracellular volume (15 L) and the intracellular volume (30 L) by the plasma milliosmole concentration, you can calculate that the number of milliosmoles in these two compartments is 4350 and 8700 respectively.

In the second column you are asked to calculate the alterations that occur if the patient loses 1 L of plasma. If the patient loses 1 L of plasma, the total volume is decreased by this amount making the new total volume 44 L. Because the lost fluid is plasma, it came from the extracellular volume, thus reducing extracellular volume from 15 L to 14 L, which changes the ratio of extracellular volume to total body volume. (No fluid is pulled from the intracellular compartment because the concentration of the extracellular compartment is not changed by the loss of plasma.) The new ratio is calculated by dividing the new extracellular volume by the new total body volume (14 L ÷ 44 L = 0.318). Although the intracellular volume remains constant at 30 L, the intracellular volume to total body volume ratio changes because the total body volume changed. The intracellular volume to total body volume ratio is calculated by dividing the intracellular volume by the new total body volume (30 L ÷ 44 L = 0.682).

Because whole plasma was lost, the concentration of the body fluid does not change and remains at 290 mOsm/kg H_2O. The total number of milliosmoles present in the body is calculated by multiplying this concentration times the new total body volume. The number of milliosmoles present in the extracellular compartment and the intracellular compartment is calculated by multiplying the milliosmole concentration by the volume of these respective compartments.

In the third column, you are asked to calculate what would happen if 1 L of isotonic saline is added to the patient's original body fluid. Obviously, this will increase the total body volume to 46 L. The isotonic saline is added intravenously to the plasma (which is part of the extracellular volume) and increases this compartment from 15 L to 16 L. Intracellular volume does not change and remains at 30 L. The ratio of the intracellular and extracellular volume to total volume is calculated by dividing the volume of each compartment by the total volume. The extracellular volume ratio equals 0.348 (16 L ÷ 46 L). The intracellular to total volume ratio equals 0.652 (30 L ÷ 46 L).

Because the added fluid is isotonic, the concentration of the body fluid remains at 290 mOsm/kg H_2O. The total amount of milliosmoles in the body is calculated by multiplying this concentration by the new total volume which equals 13,340 mOsm (290 mOsm/kg H_2O × 46 L). The number of milliosmoles in the extracellular compartment equals 4640 mOsm (290 mOsm/kg H_2O × 16 L). The number of milliosmoles in the intracellular compartment equals 8700 mOsm (290 mOsm/kg H_2O × 30 L).

The Darrow-Yannet diagram illustrating the loss of 1 L of plasma should show decreased extracellular volume with no change in intracellular volume. The concentration of both compartments should remain the same because the loss of plasma did not affect the mOsm/kg H_2O concentration. The diagram illustrating the addition of 1 L of isotonic saline should show increased extracellular volume with no change in intracellular volume. Once again, the concentration of both compartments will not change because the fluid that was added is isotonic.

The values that you have calculated reflect the rapid changes that occur when plasma volume is lost or when isotonic saline is added. Clinicians will tell you that an individual who has lost a significant plasma volume through hemorrhage will require more than isotonic saline as replacement fluid. Although isotonic saline may help solve the immediate problems caused by plasma loss, much of this fluid can shift out of the circulatory system into the interstitial space of damaged or diseased tissue, a process known as "third spacing." Fluid in this third space does not participate in normal body fluid exchange and becomes a nonfunctional part of the extracellular volume. The shift into the third space occurs because factors other than fluid tonicity are affecting the ability of the circulatory system to retain the isotonic saline. These other factors include increased capillary permeability (which is often greatly increased following hemorrhagic or septic shock) and changes in hydrostatic (or hydraulic) pressure.

Example 2: Problem

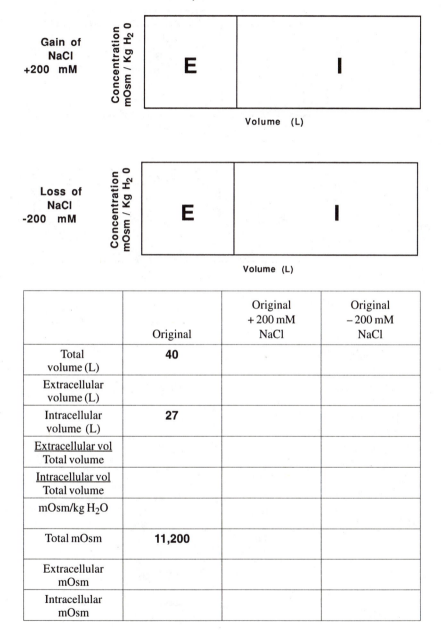

Gain of
NaCl
+200 mM

Concentration
mOsm / Kg H$_2$0

E   I

Volume (L)

Loss of
NaCl
-200 mM

Concentration
mOsm / Kg H$_2$0

E   I

Volume (L)

	Original	Original + 200 mM NaCl	Original - 200 mM NaCl
Total volume (L)	**40**		
Extracellular volume (L)			
Intracellular volume (L)	**27**		
Extracellular vol / Total volume			
Intracellular vol / Total volume			
mOsm/kg H$_2$O			
Total mOsm	**11,200**		
Extracellular mOsm			
Intracellular mOsm			

Example 2: Solution

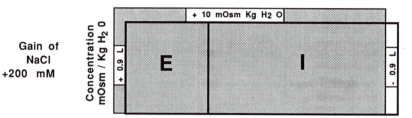

Gain of
NaCl
+200 mM

Volume (L)

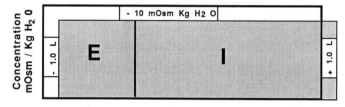

Loss of
NaCl
-200 mM

Volume (L)

	Original	Original + 200 mM NaCl	Original − 200 mM NaCl
Total volume (L)	**40**	40	40
Extracellular volume (L)	13	13.9	12
Intracellular volume (L)	**27**	26.1	28
Extracellular vol Total volume	0.325	0.347	0.30
Intracellular vol Total volume	0.675	0.652	0.70
mOsm/kg H_2O	280	290	270
Total mOsm	**11,200**	11,600	10,800
Extracellular mOsm	3640	4040	3240
Intracellular mOsm	7560	7560	7560

Example 2: Explanation

You are given that the patient's original total volume is 40 L and the intracellular volume is 27 L. By subtracting the intracellular volume from the total volume, you can determine that the extracellular volume is 13 L. The extracellular volume to total volume ratio is determined by dividing the extracellular volume by the total body volume (13 L ÷ 40 L). The intracellular volume to total volume ratio is determined by dividing the intracellular volume by the total volume.

You are given that the total number of milliosmoles is 11,200. You can determine the mOsm/kg H_2O concentration by dividing the total number of milliosmoles by the total volume (11,200 mOsm ÷ 40 L = 280 mOsm/kg H_2O). The number of milliosmoles in the extracellular compartment is determined by multiplying the mOsm/kg H_2O concentration times the extracellular volume (280 mOsm/kg × 13 L = 3640 mOsm). The number of milliosmoles in the intracellular compartment is determined by multiplying the intracellular volume times the mOsm/kg concentration (280 mOsm/kg H_2O × 27 L = 7560 mOsm).

In the second column, you are asked to calculate the change in body fluid volume and concentration that will occur if there is a gain of 200 mM of NaCl. At physiological concentrations, NaCl can be considered totally disassociated. This means that the 200 mM of NaCl, when in solution, will separate into 200 Na^+ particles and 200 Cl^- particles. Because of this, the total number of milliosmoles in the body will increase by 400 mOsm (11,200 + 400 = 11,600). You were told that solute was added, not water; therefore, total body volume remains at 40 L. The new mOsm/kg H_2O concentration can be determined by dividing the new total number of milliosmoles by the total volume (11,600 mOsm ÷ 40 L = 290 mOsm/kg H_2O). Because sodium is excluded from the intracellular space and the Cl^- will remain with the Na^+, the entire amount must be added to the extracellular compartment. This means that the number of milliosmoles in the extracellular compartment increases from 3640 to 4040 and the number of milliosmoles in the intracellular compartment remains constant at 7560. The new extracellular volume is calculated by dividing the total number of milliosmoles in the extracellular compartment by the concentration ($4040 \text{ mOsm} \div 290 \text{ mOsm/kg } H_2O = 13.9 \text{ L}$). The intracellular volume is calculated by dividing the number of milliosmoles in the intracellular compartment by the mOsm/kg H_2O concentration or by subtracting the extracellular volume from the total volume to give an intracellular volume of 26.1 L. As explained previously, the extracellular volume to total volume ratio and the intracellular volume to total volume ratio can be calculated by dividing the volume of the appropriate compartment by the total body volume.

In the third column, you are asked to calculate the changes that occur if the body loses 200 mM of NaCl. In this example, you must assume again that sodium is totally disassociated from the anion it accompanied. Thus, the loss of 200 mM of NaCl decreases the total number of milliosmoles in the body by 400 (11,200 mOsm - 400 mOsm = 10,800 mOsm). You were told that the NaCl was lost without any water. Because of this, the total volume of the patient does not change, remaining at 40 L.

The mOsm/kg H_2O concentration is determined by dividing the total number of milliosmoles in the body by the total body volume ($10,800 \text{ mOsm} \div 40 \text{ L} = 270 \text{ mOsm/kg } H_2O$). Because NaCl is excluded from the intracellular compartment, all 400 mOsm are lost from extracellular space. This means that the number of milliosmoles in the extracellular compartment decreases from 3640 to 3240. The new extracellular volume can be calculated by dividing the number of milliosmoles in the extracellular compartment by the new mOsm/kg H_2O concentration ($3240 \text{ mOsm} \div 270 \text{ mOsm/kg } H_2O = 12 \text{ L}$). The new intracellular volume can be calculated by subtracting the extracellular volume from the total volume or by dividing the number of milliosmoles mOsm in the intracellular compartment by the mOsm/kg H_2O concentration ($7560 \text{ mOsm} \div 270 \text{ mOsm/kg } H_2O$). The extracellular volume to total volume ratio and the intracellular volume to total volume ratio can be calculated by dividing the extracellular volume by the total volume and the intracellular volume by the total volume, respectively.

The gain of 200 mM of NaCl is seen in the Darrow-Yannet diagram as an increase in extracellular volume and a decrease in intracellular volume. The concentration of both compartments should increase to the same level. The loss of NaCl causes the opposite effect. The volume of the extracellular compartment decreases and the volume of the intracellular space increases. The concentration of both compartments decreases.

Example 3: Problem

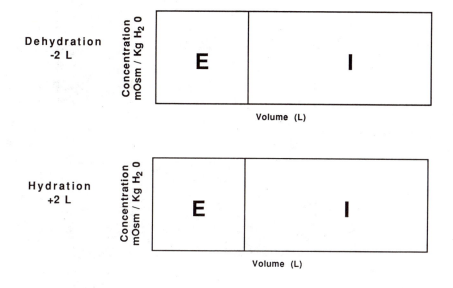

	Original	Original −2L water	Original +2L water
Total volume (L)	**42**		
Extracellular volume (L)	**14**		
Intracellular volume (L)			
Extracellular vol / Total volume			
Intracellular vol / Total volume			
mOsm/kg H_2O	**285**		
Total mOsm			
Extracellular mOsm			
Intracellular mOsm			

Example 3: Solution

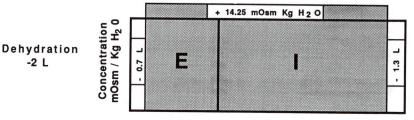

Dehydration -2 L

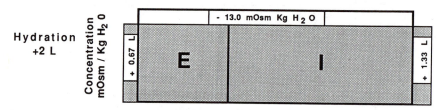

Hydration +2 L

	Original	Original −2L water	Original +2L water
Total volume (L)	42	40	44
Extracellular volume (L)	14	13.33	14.65
Intracellular volume (L)	28	26.67	29.35
Extracellular vol Total volume	0.333	0.333	0.333
Intracellular vol Total volume	0.667	0.667	0.667
mOsm/kg H_2O	285	299.25	272
Total mOsm	11,970	11,970	11,970
Extracellular mOsm	3990	3990	3990
Intracellular mOsm	7980	7980	7980

Example 3: Explanation

In this example, you are given the total body volume and the extracellular volume. By subtracting the extracellular volume from the total body volume, you can calculate extracellular volume (42 L – 14 L = 28 L). The extracellular volume to total volume ratio and the intracellular volume to total volume ratio are determined by dividing the appropriate volume by the total body volume.

You are given that the body-fluid concentration is 285 mOsm/kg H_2O. You can calculate the total number of milliosmoles in the body by multiplying the total body volume by the mOsm/kg H_2O concentration (285 mOsm/kg H_2O × 42 L = 11,970 mOsm). The number of milliosmoles in the extracellular compartment and intracellular compartment can be calculated by multiplying the volume of the appropriate space by the mOsm/kg H_2O concentration.

In the second column you are asked to determine the changes that occur in body-fluid concentration and volume after the loss of 2 L of water. Obviously, this loss decreases the total volume from 42 L to 40 L. This change should not affect the extracellular volume to total volume ratio or the intracellular volume to total volume ratio. The extracellular volume and the intracellular volume are determined by multiplying the appropriate ratio times the total body volume.

Because only water (not solute) is lost, the total number of milliosmoles in the body should not change. The new mOsm/kg H_2O concentration is determined by dividing the total number of milliosmoles by the new total volume (11,970 mOsm ÷ 40 L = 299.25 mOsm/kg H_2O). The number of milliosmoles in the extracellular compartment and intracellular compartment also should remain the same as in the original condition.

In the third column, you are asked to determine the effects that occur after an increase of 2 L of water. Obviously, the total volume of the individual increasse from 42 L to 44 L. This increase in volume should not affect the extracellular volume to total volume ratio or the intracellular volume to total body volume ratio. The new extracellular and intracellular volume is determined by multiplying the appropriate ratio by the new total body volume. Because only water and no solute was gained, the total number of milliosmoles in the body should remain constant at 11,970 mOsm. Likewise, the number of milliosmoles in the extracellular compartment and intracellular compartment should remain constant. The new concentration of the body fluid is determined by dividing the total number of milliosmoles in the body by the new volume (11,970 mOsm ÷ 44 L = 272 mOsm/kg H_2O).

The Darrow-Yannet diagram for the loss of 2 L should show a decrease in the volume of both extracellular and the intracellular compartments. The concentration of both compartments should increase to the same level.

The addition of 2 L of water should be shown on the Darrow-Yannet diagram as an increase in the volume of both the intracellular and extracellular compartments. The concentration of both compartments should decrease to a similar level.

Example 4: Problem

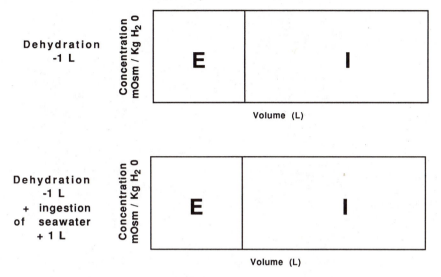

	Original	Original −1L of water	Original −1L of water +1L seawater (1000 mOsm)
Total volume (L)	43		
Extracellular volume (L)			
Intracellular volume (L)			
Extracellular vol / Total volume	.33		
Intracellular vol / Total volume			
mOsm/kg H₂O	285		
Total mOsm			
Extracellular mOsm			
Intracellular mOsm			

Example 4: Solution

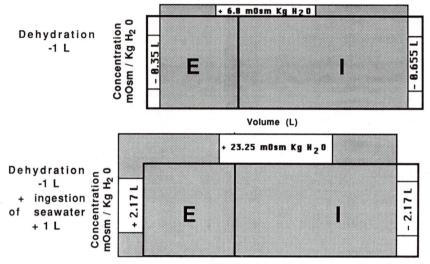

	Original	Original −1L of water	Original − 1L of water + 1L seawater (1000 mOsm)
Total volume (L)	**43**	42	43
Extracellular volume (L)	14.2	13.86	16.37
Intracellular volume (L)	28.8	28.14	26.63
Extracellular vol / Total volume	0.33	0.33	0.38
Intracellular vol / Total volume	0.67	0.67	0.62
mOsm/kg H_2O	**285**	291.78	308.26
Total mOsm	12,255	12,255	13,255
Extracellular mOsm	4047	4047	5047
Intracellular mOsm	8208	8208	8208

Example 4: Explanation

You are given that the individual has an original extracellular volume of 14.2 L and an extracellular volume to total volume ratio of 0.33. The original total volume of the individual is determined by dividing the extracellular volume by the extracellular volume to total volume ratio (14.2 L ÷ 0.33 = 43 L). If the extracellular volume to total volume ratio is 0.33, the intracellular volume to total volume must be 0.67 (1 − 0.33 = 0.67).

You are given that the concentration of the body fluid is 285 mOsm/kg H_2O. If you multiply this concentration by the total volume, you can determine that the number of milliosmoles in the total body volume is 12,255 mOsm. The number of milliosmoles in the extracellular compartment and the number of milliosmoles in the intracellular compartment can be calculated by multiplying the concentration of the body fluid by the volume of the respective compartments.

In the second column, you are asked to calculate the effect that is produced by dehydration that results in the loss of 1 L of water. Obviously, this decreases the total volume from 43 L to 42 L. This type of fluid loss should not affect the extracellular volume to total volume ratio or the intracellular volume to total volume ratio. The new extracellular volume and intracellular volume can be calculated by multiplying the appropriate ratio by the total volume. You should assume that the fluid was lost with no change in the total number of milliosmoles. The new mOsm/kg H_2O concentration is determined by dividing the number of milliosmoles in the individual by the new total volume (12,255 mOsm ÷ 42 L = 291.8 mOsm/kg H_2O). The number of milliosmoles in the extracellular compartment and the intracellular compartment should remain the same as the original condition.

In the third column you are asked to determine the effect that occurs if a dehydrated individual drinks 1 L of seawater that has a concentration of 1000 mOsm/kg H_2O. This consumption of seawater increases total body water to 43 L. The total number of milliosmoles is also increased from 12,255 mOsm to 13,255 mOsm. The concentration of the body fluid can be calculated by dividing the total number of milliosmoles in the body by the new total volume (13,255

167

mOsm ÷ 43 L = 308.26 mOsm/kg H_2O). Because most of the added solute is NaCl, you should assume that all of the milliosmoles are added to the extracellular compartment. This will increase the number of milliosmoles in the extracellular compartment from 4047 to 5047. The number of milliosmoles in the intracellular compartment remains constant at 8208. The volume of the extracellular compartment is calculated by dividing the total number of milliosmoles in the extracellular compartment by the concentration of the body fluid (5047 mOsm ÷ 308.25 mOsm/kg H_2O = 16.37 L). The intracellular volume is calculated by dividing the number of milliosmoles in the intracellular compartment by the total body concentration. The addition of the hyperosmotic seawater changes the extracellular volume to total volume ratio and the intracellular volume to total volume ratio. These new ratios are determined by dividing the new extracellular volume and intracellular volume by the new total volume.

The effect of dehydration on the Darrow-Yannet diagram is the same as that seen in Example 3, except that the volume lost in this example is only 1 L. The ingestion of 1 L of seawater causes an increase in the extracellular concentration and extracellular volume. The increased extracellular concentration causes water to shift from the intracellular compartment into the extracellular space. This shift results in a decrease in intracellular volume until the concentration of the extracellular compartment and intracellular compartment become equal.

Summary

The regulation of body fluids is important and concerns virtually every aspect of medical practice. Body-fluid shifts produced by dehydration, diseased states, trauma, and shock, to name a few, are a major concern to every member of the health-care profession. Daily intake and excretion of fluid are of interest to the veterinarian, athletic trainer, nurse, and medical practitioner alike. The points covered in this chapter represent only a brief look at the many complex factors that alter body-fluid shifts. Volumes have been written on the topic and mastery of the subject requires considerable effort and years of practical experience.

The examples in this section represent the rapid changes that occur following the loss or gain of fluid and solute. Additional factors that occur more slowly can readjust the initial changes that occur as a result of the rapid fluid shifts. For example, following hemorrhage, capillary permeability is often greatly increased, which speeds the movement of isotonic saline out of the plasma into the interstitial space. This shift can make it difficult, if not impossible, to maintain circulating volume by simply adding saline to a person in circulatory shock. In severe shock, extensive capillary damage and increased permeability allows the rapid movement of plasma proteins into the interstitial space. In such cases, even the intravenous administration of plasma proteins becomes futile. Additional problems can occur if the integrity of the sodium-potassium ATPase pump is compromised. In this situation, the cell is unable to continue pumping sodium out of the cell, which allows both sodium and water to enter the cell and increases intercellular volume.

The exercises in this chapter should help you visualize the fluid shifts that can occur; however, many additional factors must be considered before you can claim to understand fully the mechanisms involved in the maintenance of body-fluid homeostasis.

CORRECTIONS SECTION

Introduction

Throughout the examples in the text several simplifications were used to improve our ability to explain the concepts. These simplifications did not change the end result significantly, and they allowed us to more clearly explain the underlying concepts.

Now that you have a solid foundation in the concepts, the following section corrects these earlier simplifications, hopefully without confusing the issues. The first correction discusses splay. The second reviews the difference between renal plasma flow and effective renal plasma flow. Both simplifications represent fairly well understood concepts.

The latter portion of the correction section will review problems that are usually omitted from renal texts. These include concepts that are interesting but not absolutely necessary to the understanding of renal physiology.

Objectives

- Explain the difference between RPF and ERPF. How is each value calculated?

- Explain how mass balance is violated by the Fick equation.

- Construct a graph showing how the accuracy of the Fick equation is altered by urine flow rate.

- Describe why the accuracy of the extraction ratio is altered by urine flow rate.

- Explain the difference between the two clearance definitions and be able to define "cleaning clearance."

- Explain how the clearance definition used by some authors— "Clearance is the volume of plasma cleared of a compound"— is affected by the urine flow rate.

Splay

Splay was not considered in the bucket diagram examples, because ignoring splay did not significantly change the result of our calculations and simplified the math used in the calculations. However, as stated in those earlier sections, splay does alter the excretion of any compound that is transported by the renal tubules and has a transport maximum.

The transport maximum for glucose is reported to be 375 mg/min. Despite this relatively high Tm, glucose appears in the urine in most patients when the filtered load exceeds approximately 180 mg/min, which is at the renal threshold for glucose. This discrepancy is referred to as splay. Most investigators believe that splay occurs because the maximum reabsorption rate (or Tm) cannot be achieved until the amount/min of glucose being presented to the renal tubules is great enough to fully saturate the receptor sites.

Figure 10 is used to explain the concept of splay. When the filtered load is low, all of the glucose is reabsorbed (Phase I). After the filtered load of glucose reaches a point that produces initial glucose excretion, a further increase in the glucose concentration causes more glucose to be excreted and also more to be reabsorbed (Phase II). This phase continues until Tm is reached. After Tm is exceeded, any additional increase in the filtered load of glucose produces an equal increase in the amount/min of glucose excreted with no change in the amount/min being reabsorbed (Phase III).

A similar graph could be drawn for a secreted compound such as PAH. In the case of PAH secretion, the transported compound is being moved from the peritubular capillary into the tubule in a direction opposite to glucose transport. Despite this, the same concept appears to be true.

If splay had been considered in the glucose and PAH chapters , it would have been difficult to represent clearly the changes that would occur in clearance as we approached Tm. For example, when the filtered load of glucose reached 300 mg/min (glucose example 2) some glucose would appear in the urine even though we are below the Tm for glucose.

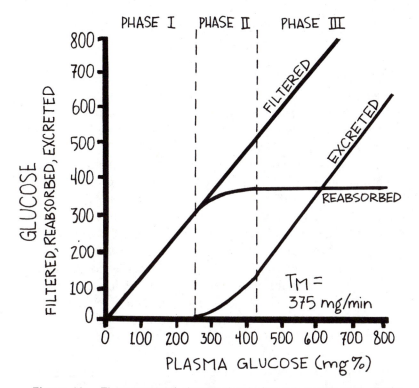

Figure 10. The amount of glucose that is filtered, reabsorbed, and/or excreted is shown on the y-axis. During Phase I all the filtered glucose is reabsorbed. In Phase II the renal threshold for glucose is exceded and glucose appears in the urine. In Phase III the Tm for glucose has been exceded and the amount of glucose excreted parallels the amount filtered as the plasma concentration continues to increase.

Renal Plasma Flow (RPF) versus Effective Renal Plasma Flow (ERPF)

In the bucket diagram examples, you assumed that when the plasma concentration of PAH is low, all the PAH that entered the afferent arteriole (site AFF) appears in the urine (site U). Most renal physiologists agree that this is true; however, not all the plasma that enters the kidney passes through an afferent arteriole (i.e., a functional nephron). Obviously, any plasma that does not pass through a functional nephron cannot have PAH removed by filtration or secretion. It is estimated that 10-15% of the plasma entering the renal artery does not pass through a functional nephron and is shunted to the renal vein. In the example illustrated in Figure 11, the shunt carries 10% of the blood that enters the kidney. Therefore, RPF equals 550 ml/min and ERPF equals 500 ml/min. Inulin is used to illustrate the effect of the shunt in this example. The concentration of inulin is the same at site 1 and at site 2; however, at the end of the nephron the concentrations differ between site 3 and site 4. No inulin is removed from the plasma passing through the shunt. When the amount of inulin shunted is added to the renal vein, the concentration of inulin at site 4 is slightly greater than the concentration at site 3. Table 3 shows several values from the example. In this example, we assume that GFR is 100 ml/min. If the Fick equation is used to determine RPF in a clinical setting, we would use the concentration at site P4 as Pv_x, which would include both the plasma that passed through the shunt and the plasma that passed by a functional nephron.

$$RPF = \frac{U_x \dot{V}}{Pa_x - Pv_x}$$

$$RPF = \frac{100\ mg/min \times 1\ ml/min}{1\ mg/ml - 0.819\ mg/ml}$$

$$RPF = 552\ ml/min$$

(Note that the RPF flow rate calculated by the Fick equation is greater than the true RPF. The reason for this inconsistency is explained in the next section.)

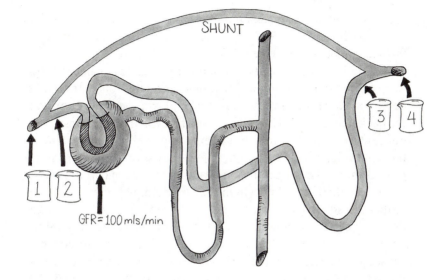

	Amount/min (mg/min)	Flow Rate (ml/min)	Inulin (mg/ml)
Site 1	550	550	1
Site 2	500	500	1
Site 3	400	499	0.802
Site 4	450	549	0.819

GFR = 100 ml/ min   Urine flow rate = 1 ml / min

Figure 11. The difference between renal plasma flow (RPF) and effective renal plasma flow (ERPF) is equal to the amount of plasma flowing through the shunt. See text for further explanation.

Mass Balance and the Calculation
Of Renal Plasma Flow and Extraction Ratio

It is not necessary to read and understand this section to understand renal function. The following is presented only for the curious who wish to pursue purity in the mathematical calculations.

The Fick equation and the extraction ratio fail to consider the flow rate of urine formed and the effect this has on the concentration of a compound in the renal vein. This can be shown most clearly by using the bucket diagrams. The calculation of RPF and Ex requires that the concentration of the compound being considered is determined in the renal vein. In correction example 1, the flow rate of urine (site U) is 1 ml/min. The concentration of inulin in the renal vein is calculated to be 0.8016 mg/ml. (In the earlier examples, you rounded off so that this small discrepancy went unnoticed.) Using the Fick equation, you can determine that RPF is 504 ml/min, which is 4 ml/min greater than the actual flow rate at site AFF. This discrepancy is caused by the slight increase in renal vein concentration caused by the excreted urine volume. If 1 ml/min of pure water is added to the renal vein to replace the fluid lost in the urine (site RV), the concentration at site RV would be 0.80 mg/ml and the Fick equation accurately would calculate an RPF of 500 ml/min.

In correction example 2, the urine flow rate is greatly increased to a rate of 10 ml/min. Although the actual RPF is held constant at 500 ml/min, the RPF calculated using the Fick equation increases to 544 ml/min. This occurred because the concentration of inulin in the renal vein was artificially elevated by the removal of more water from the plasma to form urine.

176

RPF Correction Example 1 (Inulin)

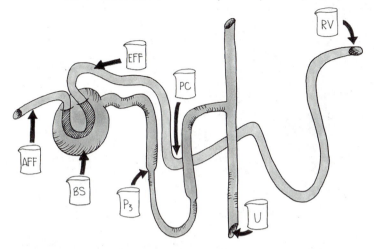

Site	Amount/min (mg / min)	Flow Rate (ml / min)	Concentration (mg / ml)
AFF	500	500	1
BS	100	100	1
EFF	400	400	1
P3	100	33	3
PC	400	467	0.87
RV	400	499	0.8016
U	100	1	100

$$RPF = \frac{U_x \dot{V}}{Pa_x - Pv_x}$$

$$RPF = \frac{100 \text{ mg/ml} \times 1 \text{ ml/min}}{1 \text{ mg/ml} - 0.8016 \text{ mg/ml}}$$

Calculated RPF = 504 ml/min

RPF Correction Example 2 (Inulin)

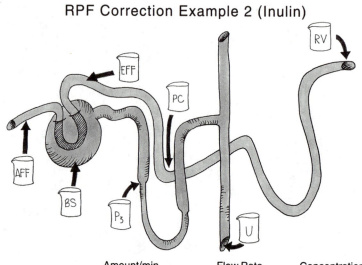

Site	Amount/min (mg / min)	Flow Rate (ml / min)	Concentration (mg / ml)
AFF	500	500	1
BS	100	100	1
EFF	400	400	1
P3	100	33	3
PC	400	467	0.87
RV	400	490	0.8116
U	100	10	10

$$RPF = \frac{U_x\dot{V}}{Pa_x - Pv_x}$$

$$RPF = \frac{10 \text{ mg}/\text{min} \times 10 \text{ ml}/\text{min}}{1 \text{ mg}/\text{ml} - 0.8167 \text{ mg}/\text{ml}}$$

Calculated RPF = 544 ml/min

As can be seen, the error in calculated RPF increases as urine flow rate increases. In most clinical cases this error is insignificant; however, the error can become rather large at high urine flow rates (Figure 12).

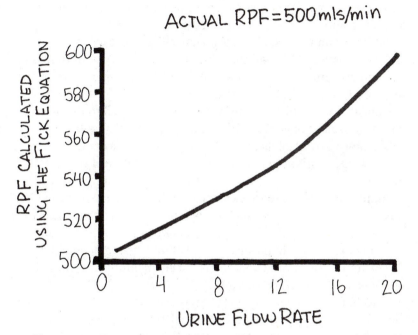

Figure 12. The error in calculated RPF increases as urine flow rate increases.

These same considerations apply to the calculation of the extraction ratio for any compound. As with the Fick equation, the extraction ratio equation requires that we determine the concentration of the compound in the renal vein. Because of this, an error appears in the extraction ratio in a manner similar to that seen in the Fick equation.

Clearance

Renal clearance often is defined as the volume of plasma "cleared" or "cleaned" of the compound being considered. This implies that a hypothetical volume of plasma appears in the renal vein that is void of the compound if the remaining plasma contained the compound at a concentration equal to that seen in the renal artery.

Inulin example 1, used to explain the RPF correction on page 177, site AFF contains 500 mg/min of inulin and 500 ml/min of fluid (i.e, each ml contains 1 mg of inulin). At site RV, 400 mg are present in 499 ml. If we could make those 400 mg appear in 400 ml of the plasma at site RV, the concentration would be equal to the original concentration seen at site AFF. In this hypothetical situation, we would now have 99 ml that would have been cleaned or cleared of in-ulin. Despite this, the calculated clearance would remain 100 ml/min.

Inulin example 2, used to explain the RPF correction on page 178, this discrepancy becomes more apparent. Obviously, as the urine flow rate increases, the discrepancy between the calculated clear-ance and the volume of plasma cleared of inulin becomes greater. In this example, the cleared volume would be 90 ml/min and the calcu-lated clearance is still 100 ml/min.

Another example of this problem is seen when we consider the clearance of glucose. If all of the filtered glucose is reabsorbed, and the kidney did not metabolize glucose, the concentration of glucose in the renal vein exceeds the concentration in the renal artery. As urine flow rate increases the concentration of glucose in the renal vein will also increase. In the case of glucose, the cleared value of plasma becomes negative.

This discrepancy led Schück to suggest that the term "clearance" be used to represent the standard equation (Equation 1) and the term "cleaning clearance" be used to represent Equation 2.

Equation 1

$$C = \frac{U_x \dot{V}}{P_x}$$

Equation 2

$$C = \frac{U_x \dot{V}}{P_x} - \dot{V}$$

In reality, no one is going to change either the clearance calcula-tion or the term itself. Because of this, it seems most appropriate to define clearance as "the volume of plasma that originally contained the amount of a compound excreted per minute." This definition sidesteps the mathematical inconsistency and presents an accurate description of the calculated value regardless of the urine flow rate.

QUESTIONS

1. The clearance equation calculates
   A. the amount of a compound excreted per minute.
   B. the volume of plasma that originally contained the amount excreted per minute.
   C. the rate that plasma is flowing through the afferent arteriole.
   D. the volume of plasma that is filtered into the glomerulus per minute.

2. The clearance of inulin is equal to GFR because
   A. inulin is freely filtered and all the filtered inulin is excreted.
   B. all the inulin entering the glomerulus is filtered into Bowman's space.
   C. the amount of inulin excreted is equal to the amount entering the glomerulus.
   D. the concentration of inulin in the plasma is equal to the concentration of inulin in the final urine.

3. The TF/P ratio for inulin changes
   A. only because water is reabsorbed.
   B. because water is reabsorbed and inulin is secreted.
   C. only because inulin is reabsorbed.
   D. because both water and inulin are reabsorbed.

4. If the TF/P ratio for compound X is greater than the TF/P ratio for inulin at the end of the proximal tubule then
   A. compound X is reabsorbed in the proximal tubule.
   B. compound X is secreted in the proximal tubule.
   C. compound X is not transported by the proximal tubule.

5. The concentration of a freely filtered compound is the same in the afferent and efferent arterioles and Bowman's space. The amount of a compound in the afferent arteriole is equal to the amount in Bowman's space plus the amount in the efferent arteriole. This is referred to as _____.

   A. clearance
   B. mass balance
   C. renal plasma flow
   D. TF/P ratio

○ 6. Filtration fraction is equal to _____.

   A. GFR/RPF
   B. clearance/GFR
   C. GFR/urine volume
   D. extraction ratio/urine volume

7. The TF/P ratio for inulin at the end of the proximal tubule is normally _____.

   A. 1
   B. 2
   C. 3
   D. 4

● 8. If the filtration fraction is 0.20 and GFR is 100 ml/min, then RPF is _____ ml/min.

   A. 5
   B. 50
   C. 500
   D. 5000

● 9. If the plasma concentration of inulin is doubled, the clearance of inulin will _____.

   A. increase
   B. not change
   C. decrease

10. If the plasma concentration of inulin is increased from 0.5 mg/ml to 2 mg/ml, the amount of inulin excreted will
    A. increase by 1.5 ml/min.
    B. increase by 2 times the original value.
    C. increase by 4 times the original value.
    D. increase by 1.5 times the original value.

11. Creatinine clearance is often used to estimate GFR in the clinical setting because
    A. creatinine is handled in the renal tubule in a manner similar to inulin.
    B. creatinine is a small molecular weight compound.
    C. creatinine is freely filtered.
    D. the reabsorption of creatinine in the proximal tubule is equal to its secretion in the distal tubule.

12. The concentration of unbound PAH _____ as it passes from the afferent arteriole to the efferent arteriole.
    A. increases
    B. decreases
    C. does not change

13. If the plasma concentration of PAH is low, the clearance of PAH is equal to
    A. the volume of plasma entering the glomerulus.
    B. the volume of plasma being filtered.
    C. the volume of glomerulus filtrate plus the urine volume.
    D. the extraction ratio divided into GFR.

14. The most likely reason your kidney secretes PAH is because
    A. PAH resembles a toxic compound.
    B. PAH cannot be filtered.
    C. PAH is often bound to plasma protein.
    D. PAH excretion helps reduce circulating nitrogen compounds.
    E. All of the above

15. The transport maximum for PAH is
    A. the maximum amount of PAH that can be filtered per minute.
    B. the maximum amount of PAH that can be secreted per minute.
    C. the maximum amount of PAH that can be excreted per minute.
    D. the maximum amount of PAH that can appear in the renal vein per minute.

16. The TF/P ratio for PAH at the end of the proximal tubule is _____ the TF/P ratio for inulin.
    A. the same as
    B. greater than
    C. less than

• 17. The clearance of glucose is normally zero because
    A. all of the filtered glucose is normally reabsorbed.
    B. the concentration of glucose in the filtrate is zero.
    C. glucose has a low molecular weight.
    D. Tm is low.

18. The TF/P ratio for glucose in Bowman's space is
    A. always 1.
    B. sometimes 1.
    C. only 1 if the plasma concentration of glucose is low.
    D. greater than 1 if the plasma concentration of glucose is low.

19. If plasma concentration of PAH is increased after the Tm for PAH is reached, you could expect
    A. both the clearance and filtered load to increase.
    B. the clearance to increase and the filtered load to decrease.
    C. the clearance to decrease and the filtered load to increase.
    D. both the clearance and filtered load to decrease.

20. If glucose reabsorption was totally blocked,
    A. the clearance of glucose would decrease.
    B. the amount of glucose excreted would decrease.
    C. the volume of urine would decrease.
    D. the clearance of glucose would equal GFR.

21. The TF/P ratio for glucose at the end of the proximal tubule is normally ____.
    A. 0
    B. 1
    C. 2
    D. 3

22. As the tubular fluid moves through the loop of Henle and distal tubule, the TF/P ratio for PAH will
    A. continue to change rapidly because PAH is secreted in the loop of Henle.
    B. continue to change only because water is reabsorbed.
    C. not change.

23. If the plasma concentration of PAH is increased to high levels, its clearance
    A. equals GFR.
    B. approaches GFR.
    C. remains constant.
    D. increases as the filtered load increases.

24. A new compound is being tested in the renal physiology lab. The concentration of the compound is found to be higher in the efferent arteriole than the afferent arteriole. From this information you can conclude that
    A. the compound is not freely filtered in the glomerulus.
    B. GFR is greater than normal.
    C. the extraction ratio for the compound is low.
    D. the extraction ratio for the compound is high.

25. The Fick equation can be used to estimate ERPF. The value calculated using this method is in error by
    A. the volume of filtrate formed per minute.
    B. the volume of urine formed per minute.
    C. a factor that increases as urine volume increases.
    D. a factor that increases as GFR increases.

26. The concentration of inulin in the renal vein will be
    A. the same as in the renal artery.
    B. greater than in the renal artery.
    C. greater than in the proximal tubule.
    D. less than in the efferent arteriole.

27. If GFR is 100 ml/min and G-T balance is two-thirds, the volume reabsorbed in the proximal tubule is _____ ml/min.
    A. 33
    B. 67
    C. 100
    D. 167

28. If the TF/P ratio for inulin at the end of the proximal tubule is 4, the G-T balance is _____.
    A. 1/4
    B. 1/2
    C. 3/4
    D. 1

29. As compared to RFP, ERPF is normally _____.
    A. 10 - 15% greater
    B. 20 - 25% greater
    C. 20 - 25% less
    D. 10 - 15% less

30. If the urine volume increases by 2 ml/min, the error in ERPF as calcuated by the Fick equation will
    A. increase by 2 ml/min.
    B. decrease by 2 ml/min.
    C. increase by more than 2 ml/min.
    D. decrease by more than 2 ml/min.

31. The concept "cleaning clearance" was introduced to correct for the volume excreted. The calculated volume of cleaning clearance will be always
    A. the same as clearance if GFR is 100.
    B. the same as clearance if urine volume is 1 ml/min.
    C. equal to clearance minus 1 ml/min.
    D. clearance minus the urine flow rate.

32. Normally, the concentration of glucose in the proximal tubule
    A. remains constant.
    B. increases because water is reabsorbed.
    C. decreases because water is reabsorbed.
    D. decreases because glucose is reabsorbed.

33. The volume of plasma flowing through the renal vein and the final urinc volume added together equal
    A. RPF.
    B. GFR.
    C. the volume in the efferent arteriole.
    D. GFR plus the final urine volume.

34. The lab reports that a patient has a plasma glucose of 400 mg/dl. The attending physician states that the patient may soon report an increase in thirst. The physician is
    A. guessing and has no logical reason to make the statement.
    B. incorrect.
    C. probably correct but could not explain the statement if questioned.
    D. correct and has a logical reason to make this assumption.

35. GFR is 100 ml/min and the TF/P ratio for inulin in the final urine is 50. This means that
    A. G-T balance is two-thirds.
    B. renal plasma flow is 500 ml/min.
    C. the urine concentration of inulin is 2 mg/ml.
    D. the final urine volume is 2 ml/min.

36. If no glucose is reabsorbed in the proximal tubule,
    A. it can all be reabsorbed in the distal tubule.
    B. it will cause glucose clearance to decrease.
    C. the amount of glucose present in the renal vein will increase.
    D. it will cause urine volume to increase.

37. The flow rate in the efferent arteriole can be determined if you know
    A. ERPF and G-T balance.
    B. GFR and the TF/P ratio for inulin at the end of the proximal tubule.
    C. GFR and the final urine volume.
    D. ERPF and GFR.

38. An investigator reports that a compound is present in the efferent arteriole at a concentration less than in the afferent arteriole. The most likely explanation is that
    A. the compound is actively transported into Bowman's space.
    B. GFR has decreased.
    C. the investigator is in error.
    D. some filtered water is reabsorbed at the efferent end of the glomerular capillary.

39. A patient has a plasma creatinine concentration of 1 mg/dl, a plasma glucose concentration of 100 mg/dl, and is excreting 1 mg/min of creatinine. The filtered load of glucose is ____ mg/min.

    A. 1
    B. 10
    C. 100
    D. 1000

40. GFR can be calculated accurately by which of the following methods?

    A. Renal plasma flow times renal fraction.
    B. G-T balance times the plasma concentration of inulin.
    C. Urine volume times filtration fraction.
    D. The urine flow rate times the TF/P ratio of inulin in the urine.

41. The amount of PAH excreted has increased but the TF/P ratio for PAH in the urine has decreased. This indicates that

    A. the clearance of PAH has increased.
    B. the filtered load of PAH has decreased.
    C. the urine volume has decreased.
    D. the plasma concentration of PAH has increased above its Tm.

42. The concentration of a freely filtered compound in the efferent arteriole can be determined if you know

    A. the flow rate and the amount of the compound in the afferent arteriole.
    B. the amount of the compound in the afferent arteriole and GFR.
    C. the flow rate in the afferent arteriole and the concentration of the compound in the final urine.
    D. the amount of the compound in the final urine and GFR.

Use the following data to answer questions 43 through 47.

The amount/min of inulin in the afferent arteriole is 500 mg/min GFR is 100 ml/min	G-T balance is 3/4 Filtration fraction is 0.2 TF/P ratio for inulin in the final urine is 200

43. The concentration of inulin in the efferent arteriole is ____ mg/ml.
   A. 0.5
   B. 1
   C. 2
   D. 5

44. The concentration of inulin at the end of the proximal tubule is ____ mg/ml.
   A. 1
   B. 2
   C. 3
   D. 4

45. The concentration of inulin in the urine is ____ mg/ml.
   A. 50
   B. 100
   C. 150
   D. 200

46. The final urine volume is ____ ml/min.
   A. 0.2
   B. 0.5
   C. 1
   D. 2

47. The volume at the end of the proximal tubule is ____ ml/min.
   A. 20
   B. 25
   C. 33
   D. 100

48. The filtered load of glucose is 600 mg/min. The Tm for glucose is 375 mg/min. This means that
    A. the patient has a below normal plasma glucose concentration.
    B. glucose reabsorption can increase by 225 mg/min.
    C. glucose is being excreted in the final urine.
    D. the patient has an elevated sodium concentration because sodium is reabsorbed with glucose.

49. A patient admitted to the hospital for treatment of edema has a plasma creatinine concentration of 5 mg/dL (normal is 1 mg/dL). Based on this information, the attending physician states that the patient has an elevated GFR. The physician is most likely
    A. correct because the filtered load of creatinine will be elevated.
    B. correct because more creatinine will be secreted.
    C. incorrect because a high creatinine level usually indicates a reduced GFR.
    D. incorrect because an elevated GFR only occurs if more creatinine is being secreted.

50. If the plasma concentration of PAH is low (so that Tm is not exceeded), the excretion of PAH will be primarily through the process of ____. If the plasma concentration is increased so that Tm is exceeded by 8 times, PAH will be excreted primarily through the process of ____.
    A. filtration, filtration
    B. filtration, secretion
    C. secretion, filtration
    D. secretion, secretion

51. If clearance of PAH is equal to effective renal plasma flow and the plasma concentration of PAH is decreased, you can expect

    A. clearance of PAH to increase.
    B. clearance of PAH to decrease.
    C. the filtered load of PAH to remain constant.
    D. the filtered load of PAH to decrease.

52. The TF/P ratio for inulin and glucose is always the same at

    A. Bowman's space.
    B. the end of the proximal tubule.
    C. the tip of the loop of Henle.
    D. the first portion of the collecting duct.

53. If RPF is constant, an increase in glomerular filtration rate causes oncotic pressure in the efferent arteriole to

    A. increase initially and then decrease.
    B. increase.
    C. decrease.
    D. not change.

54. If a compound is freely filtered in the glomerulus, its concentration in the afferent arteriole is ____ its concentration in the efferent arteriole.

    A. greater than
    B. less than
    C. equal to

55. A patient's GFR decreased from 100 ml/min to 50 ml/min. If renal plasma flow remains constant, ____ will decrease.

    A. filtration fraction
    B. glucose excretion
    C. PAH excretion
    D. urine flow

56. Secretion of PAH occurs primarily in
    A. the P1 (or S1) segment of the proximal tubule.
    B. the P2 (or S2) segment of the proximal tubule.
    C. the P3 (or S3) segment of the proximal tubule.
    D. all segments of the nephron.

57. After receiving an experimental drug, a patient is found to have an inulin clearance and PAH clearance that are equal. Decreasing the plasma PAH concentration does not change this observation. This most likely indicates that
    A. GFR is increased.
    B. PAH secretion is blocked.
    C. filtration fraction is equal to 1.
    D. the extraction ratio of creatinine is increased.

58. A drug is found that makes the ascending limb of the loop of Henle permeable to water. This drug could be used to
    A. hyperconcentrate the urine.
    B. increase glucose reabsorption.
    C. increase calcium reabsorption.
    D. increase fluid excretion.

59. The concentration of a compound in the glomerular filtrate is 1 mg/dl and its concentration in the efferent arteriole is 1.5 mg/dl. Therefore, the compound is
    A. not freely filtered.
    B. freely filtered.
    C. secreted in the proximal tubule.
    D. reabsorbed in the proximal tubule.

60. The TF/P ratio for PAH increases as the filtrate moves through the proximal tubule because
    A. water is being reabsorbed.
    B. sodium is being reabsorbed.
    C. glucose is being reabsorbed.
    D. PAH is being secreted and water is being reabsorbed.

Use the data below to answer questions 61 through 64.

The filtered load of inulin is 130 mg/min	The plasma concentration of inulin is 2 mg/ml
Filtration fraction is 0.1	

61. Renal plasma flow is _____ ml/min.
    A. 65
    B. 130
    C. 500
    D. 650

62. The extraction ratio for inulin is _____.
    A. 0.10
    B. 0.20
    C. 0.13
    D. 0.26

63. The concentration of inulin in the efferent arteriole is _____ mg/ml.
    A. 0.1
    B. 0.2
    C. 2.0
    D. 1.0

64. GFR is _____ ml/min.
    A. 2
    B. 65
    C. 130
    D. 260

Use the following data to answer questions 65 through 71.

A patient is referred to you by a local physician. In the chart that accompanies the patient, you find that:

24-hr creatinine clearance is 100 ml/min	Plasma sodium is 140 mEq/L
	Urine glucose is 100 mg/dl
Plasma glucose is 100 mg/dl (1.0 mg/ml)	Urine volume is 2880 ml/day (2 ml/min)
Plasma creatinine is 1 mg/dl	

The referring physician indicated that the patient recently started taking an experimental drug that hopefully will help control seizures. You are asked to evaluate the patient's condition.

65. The patient has a filtered load of glucose that is approximately _____ mg/min.

    A.　0
    B.　10
    C.　100
    D.　400

66. The amount of glucose being excreted is approximately _____ mg/min.

    A.　1
    B.　2
    C.　20
    D.　100

67. The clearance of glucose is approximately _____ ml/min.

    A.　0
    B.　2
    C.　20
    D.　100

• 68. The filtered load of sodium is approximately _____ mEq/min.

    A. 0.14

    B. 1.4

    C. 14

    D. 140

• 69. The patient is reabsorbing approximately_____ of the filtered glucose.

    A. 2 mg/min

    B. 98 mg/min

    C. 100 mg/min

    D. 375 mg/min

• 70. In your report to the referring physician, you should indicate that

    A. the patient is excreting glucose because GFR is extremely high.

    B. the patient is excreting glucose in the urine because the filtered load of glucose is extremely high.

    C. the patient is excreting glucose because the urine volume is high.

    D. the patient appears to have an abnormally low Tm for glucose.

• 71. A logical suggestion for treatment of the glucosuria (glucose in the urine) would be to

    A. reduce the patient's dietary intake of glucose.

    B. give an analogue of ADH to reduce urine volume.

    C. give insulin to reduce the patient's plasma glucose concentration.

    D. evaluate the experimental drug to determine if it is lowering the Tm for glucose.

Use the following information to answer questions 72 through 77.

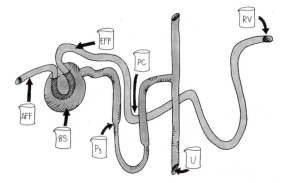

Site	Amount/min (mg / min)	Flow Rate (ml / min)	Concentration (mg / ml)	TF/P ratio
AFF	2500	500		
BS		100		
EFF				
P3				
PC				
RV				
U		1		

Points along the stylistic nephron have been identified by arrows. These arrows represent locations as follows:

AFF = afferent arteriole

BS = Bowman's space

EFF = efferent arteriole

P3 = end of the proximal tubule

PC = peritubular capillary next to the end of the proximal tubule

RV = renal vein

U = urine

In the table beneath the stylized nephron, you are supplied with several values. The values in the first column refer to the amount/min of glucose appearing at the indicated site. The second column refers to the flow rate at the various sites. The third column refers to the concentration at the various sites, and the final column refers to the TF/P ratio for glucose at the various sites. The Tm for glucose is 375 mg/min.

72. The concentration of glucose in the renal vein is approximately _____ mg/ml.
    A. 4.25
    B. 4.75
    C. 5.0
    D. 5.25
    E. 7.75

73. The filtered load of glucose is _____ mg/min.
    A. 200
    B. 500
    C. 125
    D. 2500

74. If the G-T balance is two-thirds, the flow rate at the end of the proximal tubule (P3) is _____ ml/min.
    A. 25
    B. 33
    C. 100
    D. 400

75. The amount of glucose reaching the end of the proximal tubule per minute is_____ mg/min.
    A. 0
    B. 125
    C. 200
    D. 225
    E. 500

76. The TF/P ratio for glucose at the end of the collecting tubule (urine value) is _____.
    A. 5
    B. 15
    C. 25
    D. 125

77. The renal clearance of glucose is _____ ml/min.

A. 0
B. 25
C. 50
D. 75
E. 100

Use the following figure to answer questions 78 through 83.

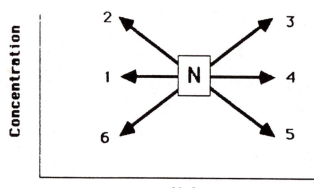

Select the arrow that best corresponds to the shift in extracellular volume and extracellular concentration that occurs with each of the conditions listed in questions 91 through 96.

78. Dehydration (loss of 1 L of water)

A. 1
B. 2
C. 3
D. 4
E. 5

79. Intravenous administration of isotonic saline

    A. 1
    B. 2
    C. 3
    D. 4
    E. 6

80. Plasma loss of 1 L

    A. 1
    B. 2
    C. 3
    D. 4
    E. 5

81. Ingestion of 1 L of distilled water

    A. 1
    B. 2
    C. 3
    D. 4
    E. 5

82. Ingestion of 1 L of seawater (1000 mOsm/kg H_2O)

    A. 1
    B. 2
    C. 3
    D. 4
    E. 6

83. The amount of sodium in the body is increased by 200 mEq.

    A. 1
    B. 2
    C. 3
    D. 4
    E. 5

Use the following figure to answer questions 84 through 90.

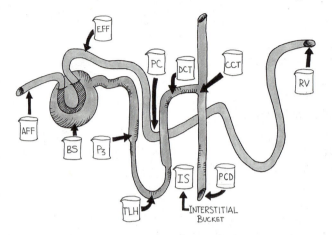

84. In a normally functioning nephron, the TF/P ratio for inulin will be similar at sites
   A. BS and P3.
   B. P3 and TLH.
   C. TLH and DCT.
   D. DCT and PCD.

85. If GFR is 120 ml/min and G-T balance is 3/4, the flow rate at the end of proximal tubule (P3) is _____ ml/min.
   A. 20
   B. 30
   C. 60
   D. 90
   E. 100

86. If the oncotic pressure in the afferent arteriole (AFF) is 20 mm Hg, the oncotic pressure at site EFF (efferent arteriole) is _____ if GFR is 100 ml/min.
   A. less than 20 mm Hg
   B. equal to 20 mm Hg
   C. greater than 20 mm Hg
   D. cannot be estimated

87. According to the passive urea recycling model, the concentration of sodium in the nephron is highest at site ____.

    A. P3
    B. TLH
    C. DCT
    D. PCD
    E. IS

88. As tubular fluid moves along the descending limb of the loop of Henle in a normally functioning kidney, its mOsm/kg H_2O concentration increases mainly because

    A. sodium enters the tubule.
    B. urea enters the tubule.
    C. water enters the tubule.
    D. sodium leaves the tubule.
    E. water leaves the tubule.

89. In the thin ascending limb of the loop of Henle, the mOsm/kg H_2O concentration decreases because

    A. sodium enters the tubule.
    B. urea enters the tubule.
    C. water enters the tubule.
    D. sodium leaves the tubule.
    E. water leaves the tubule.

90. The mOsm/kg H_2O concentration is the same at sites TLH, IS, and PCD. If this is a normally functioning kidney, you can assume that

    A. the patient is excreting a dilute urine.
    B. the patient is excreting a urine isotonic with plasma.
    C. the patient is excreting a hypertonic urine.
    D. the patient has diabetes insipidus.

Use the following data to answer questions 91 through 94.

Plasma creatinine (collected from an arm vein) is 2 mg/dl	The renal vein concentration of creatinine is 1.5 mg/dl
Urine creatinine is 200 mg/dl	Urine volume is 1 ml/min

91. GFR is _____ ml/min.

    A. 50
    B. 100
    C. 200
    D. 400

92. The filtered load of creatinine is _____ mg/min.

    A. 50
    B. 100
    C. 200
    D. 400

93. Filtration fraction is ____.

    A. 0.15
    B. 0.20
    C. 0.25
    D. 0.30

94. Renal plasma flow is _____ ml/min.

    A. 100
    B. 200
    C. 400
    D. 800

95. A patient has a urine volume of 0.5 ml/min, a urine concentration of 1200 mOsm/kg H_2O, a GFR of 100 ml/min, and a plasma concentration of 300 mOsm/kg H_2O. Based on these data, you determine that free-water clearance is _____ ml/min.

   A. +2.0
   B. -1.5
   C. -0.5
   D. +0.5

96. If the patient described in the last question is given a loop diuretic such as furosemide, you would expect the urine volume to _____ and the urine concentration to _____.

   A. increase, increase
   B increase, decrease
   C. decrease, increase
   D. decrease, decrease

97. If you gave the patient described in question 84 a maximum dose of furosemide and ADH, you would expect the concentration of urine to be approximately _____ mOsm/kg H_2O.

   A. 50
   B. 100
   C. 300
   D. 600
   E. 1200

98. A patient has a urine volume of 2 ml/min, a urine concentration of 100 mOsm/kg H_2O, a GFR of 100 ml/min, and a plasma concentration of 300 mOsm/kg H_2O. The patient has a free-water clearance of _____ ml/min.

   A. 0.67
   B. 1.33
   C. 2.33
   D. 6

99. If you gave the patient described in the last question a maximum dose of furosemide, you would expect the patient's free-water clearance to be

A. greater than +1 ml/min.
B. less than -1 ml/min.
C. approximately 0 ml/min.
D. dependent upon the plasma ADH concentration.

100. A patient has an increase in total body sodium without a change in total body water. The patient can expect intracellular volume to _____ and intracellular concentration to _____.

A. increase, increase
B. increase, decrease
C. decrease, decrease
D. decrease, increase

101. A patient drinks 2 L of distilled water. The patient's intracellular volume will _____ and intracellular concentration will _____.

A. increase, increase
B. increase, decrease
C. decrease, decrease
D. decrease, increase

102. When the Fick equation is used to calculate renal plasma flow, it overestimates the correct value because

A. the Fick equation incorrectly calculates the amount of the compound being excreted.
B. the Fick equation does not consider the increase in renal vein concentration caused by the excreted volume.
C. the Fick equation does not consider the effect of red blood cell volume on plasma volume.
D. the Fick equation is used to estimate only plasma clearance.

103. G-T balance is $2/3$ and the TF/P ratio for compound X at the end of the proximal tubule is 7.5. Based on this information you can assume that compound X is

   A. actively reabsorbed in the proximal tubule.
   B. actively secreted in the proximal tubule.
   C. passively reabsorbed in the proximal tubule.
   D. following the passive movement of water by solvent drag.
   E. neither secreted or reabsorbed in the proximal tubule.

104. Alcohol blocks the secretion of ADH. If a person with a normally functioning kidney consumes four ounces of tequila (40% alcohol), you would expect

   A. urine concentration to approach 300 mOsm/kg H_2O.
   B. urine concentration to increase because alcohol is being excreted.
   C. urine concentration to be less than the concentration of the intramedullary interstitial fluid.
   D. urine concentration to equal the concentration at the tip of the loop of Henle.

105. If a concentrated urine is being produced, the kidney is attempting to

   A. dilute the plasma concentration (mOsm).
   B. increase the plasma concentration (mOsm).
   C. increase GFR.
   D. increase urea excretion.

106. If plasma concentration of PAH is above the tubular Tm for PAH, a further increase in the plasma PAH concentration will cause

   A. the amount of PAH being excreted to decrease.
   B. the clearance of PAH to decreae.
   C. the clearance of PAH to increase.
   D. GFR to increase.
   E. filtration fraction to decrease.

107. The concentration of fluid at the tip of the loop of Henle, the interstitial fluid surrounding the tip of the loop of Henle, and the final urine is 300 mOsm. This individual has most likely
    A. consumed alcohol.
    B. received an osmotic diuretic.
    C. been given a diuretic that blocks Na^+ transport in the distal nephron.
    D. received a maximum dose of a loop diuretic.

108. Constriction of the efferent arteriole will cause GFR to _____ and renal plasma flow to _____.
    A. increase, increase
    B. increase, decrease
    C. decrease, decrease
    D. decrease, increase

109. As plasma passes along the glomerular capillary, you normally expect
    A. the concentration of freely filtered compounds to increase.
    B. the concentration of proteins to increase.
    C. the hydrostatic pressure to decrease by at least 20 mm Hg.
    D. the flow rate (ml/min) to remain constant.

110. When the plasma concentration of PAH is low (0.05 mg/ml), most of the excreted PAH is _____. When the plasma concentration of PAH is high (3.0 mg/ml), most of the excreted PAH is _____.
    A. filtered, filtered
    B. filtered, secreted
    C. secreted, secreted
    D. secreted, filtered

111. The extraction ratio for inulin is equal to
    A. renal fraction.
    B. GFR.
    C. the Tm for inulin.
    D. filtration fraction.

112. If the plasma concentration of _____ is increased by 2 times, the amount excreted is increased 2 times.
    A. glucose
    B. sodium
    C. PAH
    D. inulin

113. If glucose appears in the urine, you always can assume
    A. the filtered load of glucose is greater than the amount of glucose being reabsorbed in the proximal tubule.
    B. the filtered load of glucose is greater than the Tm for glucose.
    C. the amount of glucose being excreted is greater than the amount of glucose being reabsorbed.
    D. the reabsorbed amount of glucose is equal to Tm.

114. The reabsorption of urea
    A. is always constant.
    B. occurs only in the loop of Henle.
    C. occurs only in the proximal tubule.
    D. can change as urine volume changes.

115. If you divide GFR by the TF/P ratio for inulin at any site along the renal tubule, you will calculate
    A. urine volume.
    B. renal plasma flow.
    C. the volume of filtered fluid remaining in the tubule at that site.
    D. the volume of fluid that has been reabsorbed.

116. Intravenous infusion of hypertonic saline causes intracellular concentration to

    A. increase, because sodium moves into the cell.
    B. increase, because water moves out of the cell.
    C. decrease, because sodium moves into the cell.
    D. decrease, because water moves into the cell.

117. In the thin ascending limb of the loop of Henle, sodium is reabsorbed from the tubule and urea is secreted into the tubule. This is

    A. due to active transport of sodium at this site.
    B. due to active transport of urea.
    C. because the positive charge in the tubule forces sodium to be reabsorbed.
    D. because both sodium and urea are moving down their concentration gradient.

118. In the intermedullary region of the kidney, urea contributes 50% to the interstitial hyperosmotic gradient

    A. at all times.
    B. when the kidney is making very concentrated urine.
    C. when the kidney is making isotonic urine.
    D. when the kidney is making dilute urine.

119. The TF/P ratio for inulin at the end of the collecting duct is equal to

    A. GFR divided by urine volume.
    B. renal plasma flow divided by GFR.
    C. GFR divided by the extraction ratio for inulin.
    D. the filtered load of inulin divided by GFR.

120. Intracellular and extracellular fluid compartments always
    A. change volume in the same direction (either both increase or both decrease).
    B. change concentration in the same direction (either both increase or both decrease).
    C. increase the concentration of one compartment while decreasing the concentration of the other.
    D. decrease the volume of one compartment while increasing the volume of the other compartment.

121. Thirty minutes after the renal vein is tied off, GFR is
    A. increased because capillary hydrostatic pressure is increased.
    B. increased because hydrostatic pressure in Bowman's space is decreased.
    C. decreased because oncotic pressure in the glomerular capillary is increased.
    D. decreased because hydrostatic pressure in the glomerular capillary is decreased.

122. The concentration of a compound at the end of the proximal tubule exceeds its concentration in the afferent arteriole if
    A. the compound is reabsorbed from the proximal tubule.
    B. GFR is increased.
    C. RPF is decreased.
    D. the compound is secreted in the proximal tubule.

123. The inulin TF/P ratio at the tip of the loop of Henle is 12. The TF/P ratio for inulin will also be 12 at
    A. the glomerulus.
    B. the end of the proximal tubule.
    C. the end of the thick ascending loop of Henle.
    D. the end of the collecting duct.

Use the following figure to answer questions 124–128.

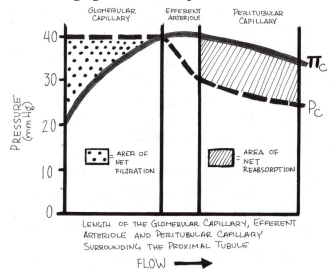

FLOW ⟶

124. According to the above graph, fluid can be expected to move

   A. out of the glomerular capillary and into the peritubular capillary.
   B. out of the glomerular capillary and out of the peritubular capillary.
   C. into the glomerular capillary and into the peritubular capillary.
   D. into the glomerular capillary and out of the peritubular capillary.

125. The above graph is used to help explain

   A. the Tm for glucose.
   B. proximal bicarbonate reabsorption.
   C. the filtered load of glucose.
   D. G-T balance.

126. If resistance in the efferent capillary is increased, GFR should ____ and the volume of water reabsorbed from the proximal tubule into the peritubular capillary should ____.

    A. increase, increase
    B. increase, decrease
    C. decrease, increase
    D. decrease, decrease

127. Filtration decreases near the end of the glomerular capillary primarily because

    A. oncotic pressure in the plasma increases.
    B. hydrostatic pressure in the plasma increases.
    C. hydrostatic in Bowman's space increases.
    D. oncotic pressure in the plasma decreases.

128. If the oncotic pressure of the plasma entering the afferent arteriole decreases by 0.25 mOsm/Kg H_2O, you should expect

    A. GFR to increase.
    B. GFR to decrease.
    C. hydrostatic pressure in Bowman's space to decrease.
    D. no change in GFR.

129. Increased concentration of sodium in the plasma always indicates

    A. an increased intracellular volume.
    B. an increased extracellular volume.
    C. a decreased total body volume.
    D. a decreased intracellular volume.

130. An increase in GFR and a decrease in RPF occurs if

    A. the afferent arteriole is constricted.
    B. the efferent arteriole is dilated.
    C. the afferent arteriole is dilated.
    D. the efferent arteriole is constricted.

131. In the absence of antidiuretic hormone, urine osmolarity is

   A. zero.
   B. less than that of plasma.
   C. equal to that of plasma.
   D. greater than that of plasma.

132. The amount of inulin that is filtered can be increased by

   A. constricting the efferent arteriole.
   B. dilating the efferent arteriole.
   C. decreasing K_f of the glomerular capillary.
   D. increasing the oncotic pressure of the plasma in the glomerular capillary.

133. Most correctly, the transport maximum of a compound refers to

   A. the rate the compound is filtered.
   B. the maximum amount of the compund that can be secreted or reabsorbed per minute.
   C. the maximum amount of the compund that can enter the final urine per minute.
   D. the rate the compound can be removed from the plasma

134. After the tubular fluid has passed through the proximal tubule but has not yet entered the loop of Henle, it is _____ when compared to the glomerular filtrate.

   A. isosmotic
   B. hyposmotic
   C. hypertonic (due to a high concentration of protein)
   D. hypertonic (due to the removal of water in the proximal tubule)

135. Most body water can be found in

   A. the intracellular space.
   B. the extracellular space.
   C. the interstitial space.
   D. the plasma.

136. Under the influence of ADH, water and urea are reabsorbed from the the
    A. proximal tubule.
    B. ascending loop of Henle.
    C. distal tubule.
    D. cortical collecting duct.
    E. medullary collecting duct.

137. As fluid moves through the proximal tubule of a normal individual, the TF/P ratio for inulin _____ while the TF/P ratio for glucose _____.
    A. increases, does not change
    B. increases, decreases
    C. decreases, increases
    D. decreases, does not change

138. A major purpose of the thick ascending limb of the loop of Henle is to
    A. concentrate the tubular fluid as it passes through this segment.
    B. decrease the volume of tubular fluid as it passes through this segment.
    C. increase the concentration of sodium in the tubular fluid.
    D. create a hyperosmotic concentration of solutes in the surrounding interstitial space.

139. After a dehydrated person drinks water
    1. extracellular volume decrease.
    2. extracellular concentration increases.
    3. intracellular volume increases.
    4. intracellular concentration decreases.

    A. 1,2
    B. 2,3
    C. 1,4
    D. 3,4

Use the following information to answer questions 140 through 143.

1. Plasma hydrostatic pressure = 50 mm Hg	3. Oncotic pressure of the plasma = 25 mm Hg
2. Hydrostatic pressure surrounding the capillary = 10 mm Hg	4. Oncotic pressure of the fluid surrounding the capillary = 0

140. These data are most likely taken from the
    A. arterial end of a peripheral capillary.
    B. venous end of a peripheral capillary.
    C. afferent end of a glomerular capillary.
    D. efferent end of a glomerular capillary.

141. The factor(s) that promote filtration of fluid out of the capillary are:
    A. 1
    B. 1, 2
    C. 1, 3
    D. 1, 2, 3
    E. 2, 3, 4

142. If K_f is equal to 8 ml/min/mm Hg, the rate of filtration across this segment of the capillary would be _____ ml/min.
    A. 60
    B. 80
    C. 100
    D. 120
    E. 140

143. If oncotic pressure of the fluid surrounding the capillary increases, then
    A. the filtration of fluid out of the capillary decreases.
    B. K_f decreases.
    C. hydrostatic pressure surrounding the capillary decreases.
    D. the filtration of fluid out of the capillary increases

144. The section of the nephron that is always relatively impermeable to water is the
    A. glomerulus.
    B. proximal tubule.
    C. descending limb of the loop of Henle.
    D. ascending limb of the loop of Henle.
    E. collecting duct.

145. A fluid sample is collected from the distal nephron by micropuncture. The TF/P ratio for compound X is determined to be 25 and the TF/P ratio for inulin is 20 at the same site. Compound X must
    A. have been secreted.
    B. have been reabsorbed.
    C. have a clearance less than GFR.
    D. have been injected intravenously.

146. A new strain of mice is shown histologically to have fewer glomerular capillaries than normal. The histologist hypothesizes that these mice would have a lower than normal rate of ultrafiltration in the kidney. If this hypothesis is true, it is most likely to occur because
    A. the filtration coefficient (K_f) is decreased.
    B. capillary hydrostatic pressure is increased.
    C. plasma oncotic pressure is increased.
    D. hydrostatic pressure in Bowman's space is increased.
    E. K_f is increased.

147. G-T balance in the proximal tubule is thought to be maintained (at least in part) by
    A. the reabsorption of fluid across the glomerular membrane.
    B. the secretion of sodium in the P1 section of the proximal tubule.
    C. the negative luminal charge seen in the P3 section of the proximal tubule
    D. the increase in plasma oncotic pressure that occurs in the peritubular capillary if GFR increases.

QUESTIONS

148. Blood flow through the renal vein is stopped by a blood clot.
A physician states this will cause the ultrafiltration rate in the
glomerulus to increase and remain elevated as long as the clot
does not dissolve. Which of the following statements could be
used to logically assess the validity of the physician's state-
ment?

A. Capillary hydraulic pressure will be decreased as long as
the clot is in place. This will cause an initial increase in
the rate of ultrafiltration in the glomerulus.
B. Capillary hydraulic pressure will remain elevated and the
ultrafiltration rate (GFR) will also remain elevated.
C. Capillary oncotic pressure will increase rapidly to offset
any change in capillary hydraulic pressure. After these
new pressures are reached, no ultrafiltrate will be formed
in the glomerulus.
D. The permeability of the glomerular capillary will
decrease because fibrin will be deposited on the
glomerular capillary.

149. Creatinine has a molecular weight of approximately 130 Daltons. Which of the following statements is most likely true
about the movement of creatinine in the kidney?

A. Creatinine does not enter Bowman's space.
B. Creatinine is freely filtered and appears in Bowman's
space at the same concentration as in the plasma.
C. Creatinine appears in Bowman's space at a greater
concentration than in the plasma because it is actively
secreted.
D. Creatinine appears in Bowman's space at a concentration
that is approximately 1/2 that of plasma.
E. The concentration of creatinine in Bowman's space
cannot be determined unless you know the oncotic
pressure in Bowman's space.

218

150. The rate of ultrafiltration in a kidney is increased. Before any data are available, a physician hypothesizes the problem is caused by increased capillary hydraulic pressure. You are asked to evaluate the accuracy of this hypothesis. Most correctly, your evaluation would state that the hypothesis

    A. is without question, totally correct.
    B. is without question, totally incorrect.
    C. may be partially correct but addtional data are needed before a definitive evaluation can be made.
    D. must be restated so that the assumptions of the scientific method are clearly indicated.
    E. cannot be evaluated because the physician was obviously guessing

151. If a compound dilates the afferent arteriole, you would expect GFR to ____ and renal blood flow to ____.

    A. increase, increase
    B. increase, decrease
    C. decrease, increase
    D. decrease, decrease
    E. not change, not change

152. The extraction ratio for PAH is highest when

    A. the Tm for PAH has not been exceeded.
    B. the clearance of inulin is high.
    C. RPF is low.
    D. renal fraction is less than 20%.

153. If active transport of sodium out of the ascending limb of the loop of Henle was blocked, which of the following will occur within 5 minutes?

    A. Inulin clearance will increase.
    B. Sodium clearance will decrease.
    C. Medullary osmotic gradient will decrease.
    D. GFR will increase.
    E. RPF will increase

154. With low ADH levels in the blood, at which of the following sites along the nephron is osmolality the highest?
    A. Fluid in the beginning of the proximal tubule
    B. Fluid in the end of the proximal tube
    C. Fluid in the tip (bend) of the loop of Henle
    D. Fluid in the beginning of the distal tubule
    E. Fluid in the end of the collecting duct

155. A substantial increase in the plasma concentration of glucose (100 mg/dl to 600 mg/dl) causes its clearance to _____. A similar change in the plasma concentration of inulin will _____ its clearance.
    A. increase, increase
    B. decrease, increase
    C. increase, not change
    D. decrease, not change

156. The amount of PAH secreted in an experimental subject could be determined by
    A. the amount of PAH excreted minus the filtered load of PAH.
    B. the amount of PAH excreted plus the plasma concentration of PAH.
    C. the urinary volume times the plasma concentration of PAH.
    D. the plasma concentration of PAH times the amount of PAH filtered.

157. The TF/P ratio for inulin
    A. increases in the collecting duct if a concentrated urine is being produced.
    B. increases in the thick ascending limb of the loop of Henle.
    C. equals 1 at the distal end of the proximal tubule because fluid is reabsorbed isosmotically in this segment.
    D. is unaffected by water reabsorption because inulin is not reabsorbed.

Use the following conditions to answer questions 158 and 159.

1. Increased hydrostatic pressure in the glomerular capillary 2. Increased oncotic pressure in the glomerular capillary	3. Increased renal plasma flow 4. Decreased renal plasma flow 5. Increased GFR 6. Decreased GFR

158. Dilation of the efferent arteriole most likely would cause

    A. 3, 6
    B. 1, 3, 5
    C. 2 only
    D. 5 only

159. Constriction of the efferent arteriole most likely would cause

    A. 2, 3, 5
    B. 3, 4, 5
    C. 2, 3, 4, 5
    D. 1, 2, 4, 5
    E. 1, 2, 3

160. You would expect the filtration of water across the glomerular capillary to be

    A. increased if hydrostatic pressure in the capillary is decreased.
    B. increased if colloid osmotic pressure in the capillary is increased.
    C. decreased if colloid osmotic pressure in the glomerulus filtrate is increased.
    D. decreased if plasma colloid osmotic pressure is increased.

ANSWERS

Question	Answer	Question	Answer
1	B	32	D
2	A	33	A
3	A	34	D
4	B	35	D
5	B	36	D
6	A	37	D
7	C	38	C
8	C	39	C
9	B	40	D
10	C	41	D
11	A	42	A
12	C	43	B
13	A	44	D
14	A	45	D
15	B	46	B
16	B	47	B
17	A	48	C
18	A	49	C
19	C	50	C
20	D	51	D
21	A	52	A
22	B	53	B
23	B	54	C
24	A	55	A
25	C	56	B
26	D	57	B
27	B	58	D
28	C	59	A
29	D	60	D
30	C	61	D
31	D	62	A

ANSWERS

Question	Answer	Question	Answer
63	C	95	B
64	B	96	B
65	C	97	C
66	B	98	B
67	B	99	C
68	C	100	D
69	B	101	B
70	D	102	B
71	D	103	B
72	B	104	C
73	B	105	A
74	B	106	B
75	B	107	D
76	C	108	B
77	B	109	B
78	B	110	D
79	D	111	D
80	A	112	D
81	E	113	A
82	C	114	D
83	C	115	C
84	C	116	B
85	B	117	D
86	C	118	B
87	B	119	A
88	E	120	B
89	D	121	C
90	C	122	D
91	B	123	C
92	C	124	A
93	C	125	D
94	C	126	A

ANSWERS

Question	Answer	Question	Answer
127	A	144	D
128	A	145	A
129	D	146	A
130	D	147	D
131	B	148	C
132	A	149	B
133	B	150	C
134	A	151	A
135	A	152	A
136	E	153	C
137	B	154	C
138	D	155	C
139	D	156	A
140	C	157	A
141	A	158	A
142	D	159	D
143	D	160	D